MIND OVER HEALTH

3in1 guide to a perfect body

(Weight loss, Muscle gain and Diet plan)

By T.K Hussain

T.K HUSSAIN

T.K HUSSAIN

To my husband

Table of Contents

Introduction

How many times have you caught yourself in front of the mirror, after showering, before dressing, and went out questioning the beauty of your body?

The process is the same: look here, pull there, I need to crumple these hips on one side, oh, I have to tighten my waist on the other, as if you were shaping your silhouette with your hands: 'my breasts could be more standing up', 'my muscles are not well built', 'I need to work out more a little…'.

This routine can be quite common.

I know much has been said about the perfection of the human body and the standards of beauty. The reality is that the synonym for the perfect body is not necessarily a thin body, but a healthy one.

After all, many thin people have very serious health problems, right?

Having a perfect body means losing fat, toning and gaining muscles, improving physical fitness, your appearance, and self-esteem, in addition to acquiring vitality and body endurance.

So, more important than losing weight at all costs, is taking care of your health so that you can feel good and willing all year round.

What makes having a perfect body hard?

Maintaining a healthy body is not an easy task, trust me, it can be very difficult especially when you need to maintain a balanced routine.

The busy and hectic routine that many people face, makes it very difficult to be able to eat properly, the amenities and comforts of technology and current life make physical exercises less frequent and uninteresting. A healthy diet, depending on the situation, is often not as accessible as well.

How this book helps

Losing weight requires a lot of discipline and dedication, but more than that, it requires understanding that it is not magic, but a process of learning, creating new habits, and a lot of patience. It doesn't happen overnight, it requires time and daily effort.

There must be an awareness that the process needs to be adequate, avoiding risky treatments, which promote very rapid weight loss, damaging your health. The weight loss needs to be a consequence of the adoption of a more regimented routine, light and healthy.

This is what I focus upon in this book, *Mind Over Health.*

In addition, I've also included a 30-day Healthy Weight Loss and Muscle Gain Eating Plan that takes the guesswork out of preparing meals that will set you on your way to your weight loss and wellness-fulfilling goals.

Can everyone have a perfect body?

If you don't try, how will you know?

I was obese in my adolescence, weighing a hundred and ten kilos.

With obesity, my self-esteem went down, and, consequently, depression, high cholesterol, anxiety, insomnia, high blood pressure, muscle pain, intestinal problems, and difficulty in concentration arose.

Time passed and I realized that only I could change that situation because the tendency was for it to get worse and worse.

'You have to lose weight' the doctor told me.

Guess what? I did it!

So yes! everyone can have a perfect body.

T.K HUSSAIN

You just need to know-how and be ready to put in all the work.

That's why this book should be your close companion.

I'm in the process of getting a perfect body.

And, I love sharing what I know!

So are you ready to start this journey with me?

Let's roll!

MIND OVER HEALTH

Chapter One

Understanding Your Body

"The body is our most archaic memory. Each event experienced leaves its deep mark on the body ". (Jean-Yves Leloup, in the body and its symbols)

Imagine this: you are about to enter a job interview. Your heart is racing, your hands are beginning to sweat, and your body is shaking all day. Yes, all of these reactions are physical and you feel them. But, have you ever stopped to think about what happens - in fact - inside to unleash all that there? Because that's exactly what we tell here.

Stress, a sedentary lifestyle, poor diet, and lack of water are everyday habits that do great harm to health. However, the body responds in the form of symptoms and malfunction. We often ignore these signs, however, they can indicate a lack of some vitamin, excess fat in the organs, or even the evolution of some diseases.

The modern routine, always full of chores, ends up taking people away from several important health activities, isn't it?

Whether preparing a balanced diet or balancing work and rest, the widespread rush causes us to neglect important choices that impact our well-being, our mind, and - consequently - our body.

Body adaptation

Here's one of the fundamental things to understand: the body is always ready to listen to you - you never spoke to it, you never tried to communicate with it. You were in it, you used it, but you never thanked it. It serves you and serves you as intelligently as possible.

Nature knows that the body is more intelligent than you, and therefore nothing important in the body is left to you, all this is left to the body itself. For example, breathing, or heartbeat, or circulation, or digestion, none of this is left to you; otherwise, you would have been in chaos long ago.

If breath control were left to you, you would already be dead. You would have no opportunity to live because you can forget about it at any moment. If, for example, you fight with someone, you will forget to breathe. At night, in a dream, you can forget that your heart has to beat. How will you remember? Do you know what work the digestive system does? You constantly swallow something and think that you are doing a great job. Anyone can swallow.

During the Second World War, it happened that a bullet hit a man in the throat. He remained alive, but he could no longer eat or drink with the help of his throat, the entire passage had to be closed. The doctors cut a small opening in the wall of his stomach that exited the tube, and he had to put food in the tube, but it was not fun. Even ice cream ... he was very angry:

"This is unbearable ... I do not feel any taste".

Then one of the doctors suggested:

"Do this: taste the food first, then put it in the tube"

And he did for forty years. First, he chewed food and enjoyed it, then put it into the pipe.

At some point in high school, you learned about anatomy, but not the truth that your body is a vessel of information, communicating with your needs and wants. You believe that your body must work for you when in fact you are complicit in your health as well as your illness. Your magician body has become mechanical, and if you want, you can even inflict violence on them when they don't do what we want them to do.

The body's communication with the mind has been turned off so gradually that there is no room for the awareness that this has happened. Like a bright light fading, the heads bow and their energy dwindle. It becomes laborious to move your body.

There is a moving paradox here: being in our bodies can seem incredibly painful. Our bodies store traumatic memories, indomitable emotions, and unfulfilled desires. But being disconnected from our bodies also means that we are separated from our hearts and souls, the very sacred source within us.

The only solution is to enter the fire of our pain, whenever and wherever you can, and learn to deal with the infinity of wisdom that your body communicates with you, all the time. Your body speaks.

Your body is your friend and not your enemy. Listen to its language, decipher its thoughts, and little by little, as you enter this book, you will realize the whole mystery of life.

It is summarized in your body. It is contained in you.

Food, diet, and nutrition

Here you will find everything you need to follow a diet and eat healthy, knowing the nutritional value of food, calories, amount of fat, and protein. Everything for a healthy life at any stage of life.

You've probably heard the common expression more than once: "We are what we eat." And indeed it is. The choice of food directly affects our health. Food is the source of building materials for our cells, tissues, and organs. It ensures the vital functions of the body, gives us energy, and even affects our mood. That is why proper nutrition is one of the most important conditions for a healthy lifestyle.

✓ Who should consider switching to proper nutrition?

- For those who want to lose weight and get rid of excess weight.
- Those who decided to take the path of a healthy lifestyle (HLS).
- Those who play sports and want to keep themselves in good physical shape.
- For those who want to avoid possible health problems caused by poor diet.
- Those who already have health problems caused by poor nutrition and must follow a sensible diet (gastrointestinal problems, cardiovascular diseases, etc.)
- For those who want to introduce themselves and their family to healthy habits.

The most common reason for switching to proper nutrition is the desire to lose weight and gain muscle. According to statistics, 54% of men and 59% of women in the world are overweight. Most often, overweight is the result of poor eating habits, eating disorders, unlimited consumption of high-calorie foods, and low physical activity. And being overweight is not just a matter of aesthetics and beauty. It is a question of the health and normal functioning of all organs in our body.

Of course, proper nutrition is a very broad concept that includes many aspects and points of view. We will give only general universal rules - they are suitable for almost everyone (with rare cases when there is a need to exclude a specific group of people). In the future, you can always optimize your diet based on the characteristics of your body and the experience of consuming certain foods.

✓ Six easy steps to proper nutrition

This step includes five simple tips to help you take the big step towards nutrition without too much theoretical immersion. Even following these simple rules, you can lose those extra pounds, cleanse your diet and train yourself to eat wisely.

The division into stages will help those who have not adhered to the principles of proper nutrition before or cannot yet afford to drastically restructure their diet. If you already have proper nutrition experience or you are a strong-willed person, then you can read the book from beginning to end and immediately start completely changing your diet.

STEP 1: Remove "food waste"

The very first step you need to take on the path to good nutrition is to eliminate so-called "food junk" from your menu, namely:

- sugar and sugar-containing foods
- white pastries and white flour products
- sausage, sausages, semi-finished meat products
- fast food (french fries, hamburgers, chips, snacks, etc.)
- sweet juices, soda, and lemonades
- mayonnaise, ketchup, and unnatural sauces

Firstly, these are foods with low nutritional value, which practically do not bring any benefit to the body. Secondly, these are high-calorie foods that are quickly stored in fat. Thirdly, most of these foods do not saturate the body, so you will constantly feel hungry and eat an excessive amount of food. By clearing your diet of this group of foods, you will already take a huge step towards proper nutrition and weight loss.

STEP 2: Eliminate alcoholic beverages

The second step involves the exclusion of another group of low-use products - alcoholic beverages. We will not now speculate about the presence or absence of harm from alcohol with reasonable restrictions, and even take into account the possible positive properties of red wine.

When switching to proper nutrition, we recommend that you give up alcohol altogether, at least for the period of weight loss.

✓ **Why it is better to give up alcohol:**
- Studies have shown that alcoholic beverages act on neurons that control appetite, which makes the body feel intensely hungry.
- Even a small dose of alcohol often provokes a food breakdown, when you, due to the loss of control, begin to "sweep away" healthy and unhealthy foods in large quantities.

- Alcohol retains water, so the next day on the scales you are virtually guaranteed to see a "gain", which is very demotivating.
- Alcohol slows down your metabolism, so your body will lose weight at a slower rate.
- Alcoholic drinks are often bundled with snacks and snacks that add extra calories.

By the way, weak alcoholic beverages cannot be classified as high-calorie foods. 100 ml of dry red wine contains 80 kcal, 100 ml of beer contains 45 kcal (but strong vodka already contains 230 kcal per 100 g). Therefore, some people allow themselves a glass of dry wine or a glass of beer once a week without sacrificing weight loss.

However, remember that in the first months of switching to proper nutrition, you are most vulnerable. Eating habits have not yet settled and the risk of breakdown is very high, so it is better to avoid provocative foods that "discourage" and relax. And alcohol is one of those.

STEP 3: Establish a drinking regime

The third step towards proper nutrition is to establish a drinking regimen, or, in other words, start drinking water. On the one hand, this step is very simple, but at the same time, it is very effective for losing weight. First, water is involved in almost all biochemical processes in the body, including the breakdown of fat. Secondly, water suppresses appetite and does not allow you to eat too much. The benefits of water in the process of losing weight are invaluable, while its energy value is 0 calories.

Train yourself to drink 1.5-2 liters of water a day (this is about 6-8 glasses of 250 ml). At first, it will seem to you that it is unrealistic to drink such an amount of water in a day, but gradually you will be able to make it your healthy habit.

- Drink one glass of water upon waking.
- Drink one glass of water before meals (20-30 minutes).
- Drink one glass of water before and after exercising.
- Drink one glass of water 30-60 minutes before bed.

In order not to forget to drink water, put yourself a reminder on your phone. There are so many convenient mobile apps that remind you to drink. Also, try to keep a bottle of water with you at all times (at work and home).

STEP 4: Set up your diet

The fourth step will be one of the most difficult, but also the most important at the same time. At this stage, many stumble, and either give up the idea of proper nutrition or slide into rigid diets. That is why, at the first stage of the transition to proper nutrition, it is better to establish at least the diet as a whole. The subtleties of the distribution of proteins, carbohydrates, and fats in the food you eat will be considered in the next chapter. So, the general diet will look like this:

- Full breakfast (7:00-8:00)
- First snack
- Lunch (13:00)
- Second snack

- Dinner (19:00)
- Late-night smoothie 1 hour before bedtime (21:00)

The time is indicated conditionally, taking into account the rise at 6:00 and departure for bed at 22:00. If you get up later or earlier, adjust the time to fit your schedule.

The main basis for proper nutrition: eat every 3 hours in small portions (200-250 g). This means you don't have long breaks between meals. Do not forget about breakfast (breakfast should be within an hour after waking up). You don't starve yourself between meals, but rather nutritious snacks. Skipping breakfast, skimpy lunches, and canceling dinners will slow down your metabolism and have a 99% chance of leading you to an eating disorder.

At the same time, your breakfast, lunch, and dinner should be full meals, and not "coffee with a cookie" or "kefir with an apple". More details about the menu will be discussed in the next chapter. But at the first stage of the transition to proper nutrition, train yourself to at least a correct and balanced diet about every 3 hours. The break between meals should not exceed 4 hours.

Such nutrition increases metabolism and speeds up the process of losing weight and staying healthy, and also provides the body with the necessary energy and nutrients. You will stop being constantly hungry and stop living with the feeling that you are on a diet.

STEP 5: Tune in to a lifestyle change

If you want not just to lose weight, but to maintain the result obtained and maintain it throughout your life, then you need to remember one more important principle of proper nutrition. Eating good nutrition should be a part of your life, not a short-term step for losing weight. Tune in to change your eating habits forever. Your body will thank you not only for a slim body but also for good health.

Many people think in this way: "Now I will sit on the right diet, get rid of excess weight, and then calmly eat whatever I want." But this is a misconception. Weight cannot be static, it changes depending on your diet. If you balance between eating well and eating haphazardly, you will gain weight swing. Kilograms will go away, and then gain again when you return to the previous diet.

The situation is similar with diets, only here everything will be much worse. Usually, the diet is low in calories, so it is very difficult to sustain it for more than three to four weeks. During this period, you may lose 3-5 kg, but most of this lost volume is not fat, but the water that goes away when you reduce the intake of carbohydrates, sweets, and saltiness. At the same time, the body adapts to a low-calorie diet, slows down metabolism, and after returning to the usual diet, it intensively accumulates fat. As a result, after the diet, you gain even more weight than you lost before.

Universal advice for losing weight: even if some fast diet seems effective to you and even if it has worked more than once, put it off right now. Sooner or later, you will still come to proper nutrition, but by that time you will already have health problems, killed metabolism, and frustration from the endless swing of weight loss and gain. Start changing your lifestyle and eating behavior, rather than go on a diet.

STEP 6: Increase physical activity

So many health problems arise from a sedentary lifestyle. Lack of physical activity causes a decrease in bone mass, muscle atrophy and weakness, a decrease in strength and endurance, and dysfunction of the spine and joints. People leading a sedentary lifestyle very often face problems such as osteochondrosis, osteoporosis, sciatica, hernia, scoliosis, as well as several cardiovascular diseases.

Therefore, regular exercise is one of the most important healthy habits. This will not necessarily be training in the gym or some other intense load, which has some restrictions, including excess weight. It can be regular exercises, yoga, dancing. , sports games, cycling. The main thing is that this physical activity pleases you. You can start exercising at home for at least 10-20 minutes a day.

If you have contraindications for physical education or you have a lot of excess weight (for example, you need to lose more than 30 kg), then start at least with a regular walk for 30-40 minutes a day. This can be walking in the morning before work or in the evening after. You can buy a fitness bracelet and track the number of steps taken. Start with 5,000 daily steps and add 1,000 steps every week. You will feel how physical activity gives energy, strength, and vitality.

The myth about exercise

Regular physical exercise is essential to achieve a good quality of life. The World Health Organization (WHO) recommends a weekly minimum of 150 minutes of light or moderate activity or 75 minutes of more intense activity.

The benefits of exercising go beyond weight loss and also contribute to raising self-esteem, preventing osteoporosis, and combating obesity - a risk factor for various diseases.

However, the practice of a physical activity is surrounded by several mysteries, such as which types of exercises are most suitable or regarding schedules and intake of supplements.

When it comes to healthy and lasting weight loss, a balance between physical exercise and healthy eating is necessary.

See below what is a myth and what is true about the weight loss process.

- **Exercises are the best way to lose weight**

#MYTH. It is no use practicing physical exercises and eating incorrectly. To achieve a balance between these two factors, much is said about the 80/20 or 70/30 ratio, respectively, for diet and exercise.

However, experts claim that there are no magic formulas. Weight loss only works with a "Negative Energy Balance", which consists of consuming fewer calories and/or increasing energy expenditure through exercise and daily activities.

- **Bodybuilding turns fat into muscle**

#MYTH. It is impossible to build muscle from fat because they are different tissues. The adipose tissue (fat) is located under the skin, between the muscles, and around the internal organs. Since muscle tissue (muscle) is found throughout the body.

Weight training is strength training. By practicing it, we improve the conditioning of muscles and expend calories, which helps to reduce fat tissue. However, aerobic exercise is considered the best exercise to burn fat.

- **People who start working out can gain weight**

#TRUTH. But don't be alarmed by the answer. Weight exercises help in gaining lean mass, i.e. muscles. It is normal for this type of training to generate weight gain, which is often visually noticeable.

With the growth of muscles, consequently, body fat decreases and the body becomes more defined and more beautiful. When starting a training routine, it is recommended to take the main body measures to follow the evolution.

- **Fasting training helps you lose weight faster**

#MYTH. When we wake up, we usually go six to eight hours without eating and with low blood glucose. Glucose is the body's main source of energy and without a supply of carbohydrates, the body uses muscle mass as an energy source.

Training without eating can even cause the individual to lose fat, but this is an extremely dangerous option. During exercise, there is an increased risk of hypoglycemia, which can cause malaise, headaches, and nausea.

- **You should not drink water during exercise**

#MYTH. When we sweat excessively, the body loses water and electrolytes (a combination of sodium, potassium, and other nutrients). The intensity of the exercises and the lack of fluid can cause dehydration, characterized by symptoms such as dizziness, muscle spasms, and kidney problems.

Therefore, hydration is important and indispensable during physical exercise. Whether through the consumption of water, coconut water, isotonic drinks, or teas, these fluids help to keep the body healthy and prevent injuries.

- **Green tea speeds up metabolism**

#TRUTH. As already explained, teas can be consumed during exercise. These drinks are known for their therapeutic power, as they have powerful antioxidant agents in their composition that protect the body and prevent disease.

Green tea has thermogenic ingredients, which causes the metabolism to work at a fast pace and spend more calories. This tea also promotes the oxidation of increased fat, generating a reduction in fat mass and body weight.

- **Sit-ups dry the belly**

#MYTH. These exercises strengthen the muscles of the abdominal region. However, only they do not burn localized fat. To dry the belly, it is necessary to invest in a balanced diet and cardiorespiratory and/or aerobic exercises.

Another exercise that helps define the abdomen is the plank, which can be done by beginners or experienced people, at the gym or home. This exercise works several muscles at the same time, also strengthening the muscles of the lower back and pelvic area

And now that you know all the myths and truths about physical exercise, what is missing is to start working? Believe me, this is the only effective way to lose weight and stay healthy permanently.

Let's delve into Food and Calorie Count in the next chapter.

My heart thanks you!

Chapter Two

Your Food and Calories

Healthy eating is a recurring theme in our daily lives. Diets and more diets come up all the time to help us lose weight, which often doesn't. One of the biggest causes is the lack of knowledge about what we can eat, or simply knowing how many calories the food we are going to eat at lunch, for example, with the plate in front of us.

Contrary to what you might think, calories aren't just there to ruin our lives! Whether we like it or not, we need it: calories provide us with the energy we need every day to cover our body's expenses. Because yes, even if we often skip sports lessons, our body burns calories even while sleeping! To lose weight effectively, you must therefore ensure that you balance the number of calories consumed and the number of calories expended throughout the day.

On the other hand, you are probably wondering why your girlfriend or your sweetheart can eat twice as much as you without putting on weight. Because we don't have the same calorie needs. They depend on our age, our sex, our morphology, our physical activities, the time of day when the calories were consumed and many other variables.

This is why it is useless to start a diet or to set a quota of calories to consume per day without really knowing your own caloric needs.

Calorie count

A calorie is the amount of energy that a food provides to the body to perform its vital functions.

Every day, your body manages the activities of all of its cells and makes sure that they are receiving enough energy to carry out their tasks.

If you do not take in enough calories, your body will use your energy reserves to provide priority cell activities and you will lose weight. If, on the contrary, you ingest more than necessary, the excess calories will be stored as fat.

To know the total amount of calories a food has to read the label and take into account the amount of protein, carbohydrates, and fat, calculating the total calories as follows:

- For each 1g of carbohydrates: add 4 calories;
- For each 1g of protein: add 4 calories;
- For each 1g of fat: add 9 calories.

It is important to remember that other components of food, such as water, fibers, vitamins, and minerals have no calories and, therefore, do not provide energy, however, they are extremely important for other biological processes.

Calculating your calorie count

To know how many calories you should eat per day it is important to make some calculations since the value will vary according to age, current weight, sex, and height.

Your Calorie needs to depend on several factors:
• **Your age**
The amount of calories your body uses when you sleep or move around (basal metabolic rate) decreases by 2% to 3% every 10 years. And the fall accelerates around 40 years for men and 50 years for women ...
For example, children have a basal metabolism twice as high compared to their body weight as adults. And a 50-year-old woman needs about 140 Calories less each day than a 30-year-old woman.

• **Your weight and height**

The fewer cells you have to feed, the less energy your body needs to function well, both vertically and horizontally. Thus, for the same size, a man of 80 kg will consume daily about 300 Calories more than a man of 60 kg to maintain his weight.

• Your level of physical activity
Getting moving doesn't just help you spend your energy. At rest, muscles require more energy than fat mass. Do you play tennis three times a week? Well, sitting behind your desk, you burn more calories than someone your stature and age, but sedentary. A double expense!

• Your gender
Men have more muscle mass and a larger body surface area than women, so they have higher energy needs.
Other factors can increase or decrease your energy needs: pregnancy, breastfeeding, the secretion of certain hormones, undernourishment, ambient, and body temperature as well as heredity.

Also, the daily caloric value must be taken into account by each person, whether the goal is to gain weight or lose weight.

1. Direct Method

There are several ways to calculate the calorie requirement for a day, however, the easiest is the direct method, which is done as follows:

- To lose weight - multiply 20 or 25 by the current weight
- To maintain weight - multiply 25 or 30 by the current weight

- To put on weight - multiply 30 or 35 by the current weight

For example, a person who weighs 50 kg and wants to maintain his weight, must multiply 25 x 50 or 30 x 50 and, without fear of gaining weight, can eat between 1250 and 1500 calories per day.

2. Calorie budget

You are a woman, between 18 and 40 years old:

- You do not practice any physical activity: you need around 1900 calories per day.

- You are active: you need around 2150 calories per day.

- You are a great athlete: you need around 2,500 calories.

You are a woman over 40:

- You do not practice any physical activity: you need around 1750 calories per day.

- You are active: you need around 2000 calories per day.

- You are a great athlete: you need around 2350 calories per day.

You are a man, between 18 and 40 years old:

- You do not practice any physical activity: you need around 2350 calories per day.

- You are active: you need around 2650 calories per day.

- You are a great athlete: you need around 3250 calories.

You are a man over 40:

- You do not practice any physical activity: you need around 2200 calories per day.

- You are active: you need around 2450 calories per day.

- You are a great athlete: you need around 3050 calories per day.

For pregnant and breastfeeding women, you will need more calories per day: count around 340 calories for a pregnant woman from her second trimester of pregnancy, and around 330 calories for a breastfeeding woman.

Warning!

When you calculate a person's calorie needs, you make an estimate. His actual needs may therefore be lower or higher than this figure. That's why it's always best to listen to your hunger and fullness signals, which are the best indicators of how much energy your body needs.

3. Alorie counting algorithm

STEP 1: Calculate your base metabolic rate

Each of us, depending on weight, activity, and age, requires a different amount of food. To find out the exact figure, you need to use the Harris-Benedict formula:

- Women: BMR = 9.99 * weight (in kg) + 6.25 * height (in cm) - 4.92 * age (number of years) - 161

- Men: BMR = 9.99 * weight (in kg) + 6.25 * height (in cm) - 4.92 * age (number of years) + 5

Where BMR is the basal metabolic rate

STEP 2: Determine Daily Activity

The resulting base metabolic rate (BMR) figure must be multiplied by the physical activity ratio:

- 1.2 - minimal activity (lack of physical activity, sedentary work, minimum movement)
- 1.375 - Slight activity (light training or walking, little daily activity during the day)
- 1.46 - average activity (training 4-5 times a week, good activity during the day)
- 1.55 - activity above average (intense training 5-6 times a week, good activity during the day)
- 1.64 - increased activity (daily training, high daily activity)
- 1.72 - high activity (daily ultra-intense training and high daily activity)
- 1.9 - very high activity (usually we are talking about athletes during the period of competitive activity)

Note! When choosing a coefficient, it is better to focus on the overall activity during the day. For example, if you train every day for 30-45 minutes, but at the same time you have a sedentary lifestyle, then you do not need to take a coefficient greater than 1.375. One workout, even the most intense, does not compensate for the lack of activity during the day.

STEP 3: calculate the result

So, by multiplying your base metabolic rate (BMR) by your physical activity ratio, we get your calorie intake. Eating within this norm, you will neither lose weight nor gain weight. This is the so-called calorie intake for weight support.

BMR * Physical Activity Rate = Calorie Allowance for Weight Support.

If you want to lose weight, then 15-20% must be subtracted from the resulting product (this will be food with a calorie deficit). If you are working on muscle growth, then you need to add 15-20% (this will be a diet with a surplus of calories). If you are at the "weight maintenance" stage, then leave the resulting figure unchanged.

With a little excess weight, we recommend calculating the daily calorie intake with a 15% deficit. If you need to get rid of> 10 kg, we recommend calculating with a 20% deficit. With a lot of excess weight, if you need to get rid of> 40 kg, you can take a deficit of 25-30%.

EXAMPLE:

Woman, 30 years old, weight 65 kg, height 165 cm, and physical activity 3 times a week:

- BMR = 9.99 * 65 + 6.25 * 165 - 4.92 * 30 - 161 = 1372
- Calories to maintain weight = 1372 * 1.375 = 1886.5 kcal

- Calorie norm with a deficit = 1886 - (1886 * 0.2) = 1509 kcal

In total, we get 1450-1550 kcal - this is the daily rate for losing weight. Focusing on this figure, you need to keep a daily calorie count for your menu.

✓ **The importance of the right number of calories per day to lose weight**

When it comes to weight loss, it's all about balance. Calculating the right number of calories per day needed to lose weight is an essential step.

Here are the 3 possible situations:

- the energy intake is equal to the energy requirement: the weight remains stable
- the energy intake is lower than the energy requirement: there is weight loss
- energy intake is greater than energy requirement: there is weight gain

Be careful, however, that the energy deficit must not be too great at the risk of causing nutritional deficiencies and harmful adaptation mechanisms. Indeed, below a certain number of calories, the body protects itself by saving its energy and by storing more calories ingested. As a result, weight loss becomes more and more difficult and the yo-yo effect inevitable.

Food to eat

Do you know the "zero calories" diet? According to this theory, by choosing to consume foods that are low in calories, the energy you burn by eating those foods exceeds the number of calories they contain. This means that the number of calories needed to consume these foods exceeds the number of calories in the foods you eat. It is difficult to determine if this theory is correct. But what's for sure is that low-calorie foods can help you shed those extra pounds. g). To lose weight, you must find good eating habits. A varied and balanced diet involves the consumption of foods beneficial to your health (fruits, vegetables, starchy foods, fish, etc.) and a reduction in fatty foods (cold meats, butter, cream, etc.), sweet foods (pastries, sweet drinks…), and savory (appetizer cakes, crisps…).

According to the National Health Nutrition Program (PNNS), it is recommended to have a varied and balanced diet to consume:

- **Proteins (meat, eggs, and fish): once or twice a day**

To lose weight, favor lean meats such as chicken, turkey, veal, etc., steamed, grilled fish.

- **Dairy products: 1 to 2 servings/day**

Prefer low-fat unsweetened yogurts and cottage cheese. Preferably consume low-fat cheeses.

- **Starchy foods: at every meal**

Opt for wholemeal bread, wholemeal pasta, brown rice, and cereals. Rich in nutrients and fiber, they have a satiating effect.

- **Fruits and vegetables: 5 per day at least**

The vegetables can be eaten at will, cooked, in soup, or raw vegetables. Choose seasonal vegetables which will allow you to cook varied. During a diet, favor low-calorie fruits according to the seasons.

- **Water: approximately 1.5 liters per day**

Water is the drink par excellence to keep the figure! Water helps to hydrate and helps eliminate waste from the body. It also fights against water retention.

Here are some tips for lasting and healthy weight loss:

- Eat slowly, calmly, and take the time to chew well
- Do not skip meals
- Maintain sufficient hydration, at least 1.5 liters of water per day
- Always favor seasonal and fresh plants
- Give preference to whole grains and loaves of bread
- Avoid sugar and salt, favor natural sweeteners and spices to give flavor
- Systematically include a good portion of raw vegetables or cooked vegetables at each meal
- Favor simple, homemade cooking and avoid the purchase of ready-made meals

Calorie table of the most served foods

Food	Amount	Calories
Coffees, teas, and juices		
Green coconut water	1 cup of 240 ml	62
Coffee with sugar	1 cup of 50 ml	33
Coffee without sugar	1 cup of 40 ml	3
Sugar cane juice	1 cup of 240 ml	202
Natural pineapple juice	1 cup of 240 ml	100
Natural acerola juice	1 cup of 240 ml	36
Natural apple juice	1 cup of 240 ml	154
Natural Mango Juice	1 cup of 240 ml	109
Natural melon juice	1 cup of 240 ml	60
Natural green corn juice	1 cup of 240 ml	271
Natural strawberry juice	1 cup of 240 ml	39
Natural peach juice	1 cup of 240 ml	77
Fresh tomato juice	1 cup of 240 ml	27
Alcoholic beverages		
Brandy	½ cup - 120 ml	277
Beer	1 can of 350 ml	147
Light beer	1 can of 360 ml	148

Champagne	1 125 ml bowl	85
Draft beer	1 tulip of 300 ml	180
Whiskey	1 dose of 100 ml	240
Sweet white wine	1 125 ml bowl	178
Dry white wine	1 125 ml bowl	107
Rose wine	1 125 ml bowl	93
Dry red wine	1 125 ml bowl	107
Vodka	1 cup of 20 ml	48
Soft drinks and energy drinks		
Coke	1 can of 350 ml	137
Coca-Cola Light	1 can of 350	1.5
Fanta	1 can of 350 ml	189
Fanta Diet	1 can of 350 ml	15
Sports Drink lemon	2 tablespoons (20g)	51
Sprite	1 can of 350 ml	115
Meat		
Roasted rump	2 slices (150g)	301
Fried rump	2 slices (100g)	235
Homemade meatball	1 unit (30g)	61
Chicken meatballs	1 unit (25g)	54
Turkey meatball	1 unit (25g)	46
Roasted chicken thighs	2 units (100g)	109
Baby beef	1 unit (100g)	120
Sliced bacon	1 slice (10g)	54

Fried bacon	2 cubes (30g)	198
Pork chop	1 unit (100g)	337
Pork chop	2 units (100g)	483
Chicken thigh	1 unit (100g)	144
Roasted chicken leg with skin	1 unit (100g)	110
Roasted chicken leg without skin	1 unit (100g)	98
Cooked chicken leg	1 unit (100g)	120
Termite	2 slices (150g)	375
Fried beef liver	1 slice (100g)	210
Chicken liver	1 tablespoon (25g)	35
Chicken fillet	2 fillets (100g)	101
Filet mignon	1 slice (100g)	140
Bovine Hamburger	1 unit (56g)	116
Pepperoni hamburger	1 unit (56g)	149
Chester hamburger	1 unit (56g)	105
Chicken hamburger	1 unit (96g)	179
Roasted ox lizard	3 slices (100g)	170
Piglet	2 pieces (170g)	308
Boiled beef tongue	2 pieces (100g)	287
Roasted loin	1 slice (100g)	272
Mummy	1 slice (100g)	141
Soft crumb core	1 fillet (100g)	120
Chicken gizzards	1 saucer (100g)	78

Cooked muscle	3 pieces (100g)	180
Roast ox duckling	3 slices (100g)	200
Chicken breast without the skin	1 fillet (100g)	100
Shank Pork Roast	1 slice (100g)	196
Peru	2 fillets (100g)	155
Rump steak	1 slice (100g)	287
Frog	1 unit (200g)	128
Salted pork tail	3 units (100g)	426
roast beef	1 slice (50g)	83
Tend	4 slices (100g)	210
Embedded		
Turkey banquet	1 slice (10g)	13
Ripe sliced cup	1 slice (6g)	22
Pepperoni sausage	1 serving (100g)	300
Chicken sausage	1 serving (100g)	166
Smoked turkey sausage	1 serving (100g)	148
Tuscan sausage	1 serving (100g)	255
Black pudding	1 serving (100g)	258
Smoked turkey breast	1 slice (15g)	14
Baked ham	1 slice (15g)	18
Raw ham	1 slice (15g)	54
Parsley	1 unit (40g)	120
Hot Dog Sausage	1 unit (50g)	115
Sausage	1 slice (10g)	30

Fishes and seafood		
Cooked anchovy	1 fillet (100g)	118
Breaded anchovy	1 fillet (100g)	210
Raw tuna	1 piece (100g)	146
Cooked cod	1 serving (100g)	100
Cooked dogfish	1 piece (100g)	129
Boiled shrimp	1 serving (100g)	82
Fried shrimp	1 serving (100g)	310
Crab Shell	1 unit	250
Crab Cone	1 unit (200g)	413
Golden	1 piece (100g)	88
Cooked Haddock	1 fillet (100g)	100
Lobster cooked without sauce	1 unit (200g)	196
Roasted or grilled sole	1 fillet (100g)	90
Cooked squid	1 tea saucer (100g)	93
Fried squid breaded	1 tea saucer (100g)	373
Cooked seafood	1 cup of tea (100g)	96
Cooked mussels	½ cup of tea (100g)	79
Baked boyfriend	1 fillet (100g)	122
Oysters	3 units (100g)	81
Raw fish roe	1 serving (100g)	125

Cooked hake	1 fillet (100g)	97
Painted grilled	1 piece (200g)	208
Raw octopus	1 cup of tea (100g)	64
Sea Bass	1 piece (100g)	72
Roasted or grilled salmon	1 piece (100g)	292
Raw salmon	1 fillet (100g)	211
Grilled sardines	1 unit (33g)	97
Sardines in edible oil	4 units (100g)	174
Canned sardines with olive oil	3 units (100g)	298
Cooked Mullet	1 piece (100g)	204
Roasted or grilled trout	1 unit (200g)	378
Biscuits and cookies		
Water and salt	1 unit	32
Butter biscuit	1 serving (100g)	500
Whole wheat biscuit	1 unit (15g)	28
Champagne	1 unit	40
Cream cracker	1 unit	31
Milk	1 unit	24
Mary	1 unit	25
Salted sticks	100g	383
Stuffed chocolate	1 unit	72

Stuffed strawberry	1 unit	73
Chocolate wafer	1 unit	41
Bullets		
Milk caramel	1 unit	21
Average gum	1 unit	18
Halls	1 unit	19
Halls diet	1 unit	8
Cakes		
Homemade carrot cake	1 slice (50g)	135
Carrot cake with chocolate icing	1 slice (50g)	371
Chocolate Cake	1 slice (50g)	171
Homemade cornmeal cake	1 slice (50g)	310
Orange cake	1 slice (50g)	173
Sponge cake	1 slice (50g)	268
Coconut cake	1 slice (50g)	186
Chocolates		
Aerated to milk	1 unit (30g)	167
Alpine Milk Chocolate Bonbon	1 unit (13g)	71
Semisweet chocolate	1 unit (200g)	1074
Soluble chocolate powder	1 tablespoon (6g)	22
Black Diamond	1 unit (30g)	156

White chocolate	1 unit (30g)	170
White gold	1 unit (21.5g)	114
Truffles	1 unit (20g)	89
Candy		
Peanuts with chocolate	1 tablespoon (40g)	140
Sweet rice	1 serving (100g)	164
Girl spit	1 cup (150g)	615
Caramel Banana	1 unit	140
Banana raisin	1 unit (15g)	28
Chocolate bomb	1 unit (80g)	187
Chocolate bomb with chocolate icing	1 large	296
Pumped	1 unit (30g)	91
Condensed milk dessert with cashews	1 unit (12g)	102
Caramel syrup	1 tablespoon (20g)	55
Chocolate syrup with milk	1 tablespoon (20g)	109
Caramel icing	1 tablespoon (15g)	156
Cherry cover	1 tablespoon (15g)	147
Chocolate cover	1 tablespoon (15g)	128

White cocada	1 unit	55
Peanut butter	1 dessert spoon (15g)	88
Marshmellow cream	1 tablespoon (15g)	158
Soft Banana Candy	1 tablespoon (20g)	46
Milk sweet	1 slice (50g)	158
Veneer with cream	1 slice (50g)	704
Raspberry in syrup	1 tablespoon (25g)	29
Guava jelly	1 dessert spoon (15g)	30
Strawberry jam	1 dessert spoon (15g)	39
Brown icing	1 slice (100g)	270
Honey with propolis	1 tablespoon (20g)	65
Bee honey	1 tablespoon (20g)	62
Chocolate mousse	1 cup (150g)	333
Peanut candy	1 unit (30g)	114
Peach in syrup	1 unit (100g)	81
Homemade rice pudding	1 serving (100g)	230
French toast	3 slices (100g)	445
Dream	1 unit (85g)	573
Gelatin		

Pineapple	1 serving (100g)	68
Cherry	1 serving (100g)	68
Raspberry	1 serving (145g)	68
Lemon	1 serving (100g)	68
Strawberry	1 serving (100g)	68
Grape	1 serving (100g)	68
Ice creams		
Coconut milk	1 unit	94
Strawberry milk	1 unit	123
Banana split	1 cup	843
Vanilla Milkshake	1 cup (290ml)	336
Chocolate Milk Shake	1 cup (300ml)	380
Chocolate dough ice cream strawberry and coconut	1 ball (40g)	75
Lemon Dough Ice Cream	1 ball (40g)	62
Sweeteners and condiments		
Refined white sugar	1 teaspoon (10g)	40
Brown sugar	1 teaspoon (10g)	36
Caper without olive	1 teaspoon (6g)	two
Garlic	1 tooth	7
Broth	1 tablet (12g)	33
Chicken broth	1 tablet (12g)	35

Raw onion	1 tablespoon (20g)	6
Green smell	1 pack	4
Curry	1 coffee spoon (6g)	23
Tomato extract	1 tablespoon (20g)	14
Ketchup	1 tablespoon (15g)	20
Coconut milk	½ cup (120ml)	132
Red pepper sauce	1 teaspoon (6g)	two
English sauce	1 tablespoon (15g)	5
Mustard	1 teaspoon (10g)	8
Paprika	1 teaspoon (6g)	20
Black pepper	1 teaspoon (6g)	1
Refined white salt	1 teaspoon (6g)	0
Vinegar	1 tablespoon (15g)	3
Creams and sauces		
Mango chutney	1 tablespoon (20g)	82
Mayonnaise	1 tablespoon (20g)	141
Sweet and sour sauce	1 tablespoon (20g)	31
Yogurt broth	1 tablespoon (15g)	21

Rose sauce	1 tablespoon (15g)	135
Homemade Tomato Sauce	1 tablespoon (15g)	10
Fats and oils		
Palm oil	1 tablespoon (10g)	89
Olive oil	1 tablespoon (10g)	90
Chicken lard	1 tablespoon (20g)	126
Hydrogenated vegetable fat	1 tablespoon (20g)	180
Butter with salt	1 tablespoon (10g)	77
Margarine	1 teaspoon (10g)	74
Cotton oil	1 tablespoon (10g)	90
Peanut oil	1 tablespoon (10g)	90
Canola oil	1 tablespoon (10g)	90
Cod liver oil	1 tablespoon (13g)	130
Sesame oil	1 tablespoon (10g)	90
Sunflower oil	1 tablespoon (10g)	90
Corn oil	1 tablespoon	90

	(10g)	
Fish oil	1 tablespoon (10g)	90
Soy oil	1 tablespoon (10g)	90
Fresh and dried fruits		
Avocado	1 serving (100g)	177
Pineapple	1 slice (80g)	50
Acerola	1 unit (12g)	4
Plantain	1 unit (100g)	117
Raw silver banana	1 unit (65g)	55
cashew	1 unit (100g)	37
Sugar cane	1 slice (100g)	64
Chopped cashews	1 cup of tea (150g)	835
Cherry	1 serving (100g)	97
Freshly grated coconut	1 tablespoon (20g)	50
Ripe fig	1 unit (50g)	68
Raspberry	1 tablespoon (20g)	12
Red guava	1 unit (100g)	43
Kiwi	1 unit	46
Orange	1 unit	46
Lemon	1 unit	12
Green apple	1 unit (130g)	79
Red Apple	1 unit (130g)	85

Ripe papaya	1 slice (100g)	36
Mango	1 unit (350g)	230
Common passion fruit (pulp)	1 unit (50g)	28
watermelon	1 slice (100g)	24
Melon	1 slice (70g)	19
Strawberry	9 units (100g)	43
Nuts	1 unit (10g)	71
Raw pear	1 unit (110g)	68
Dried pear	1 cup of tea (150g)	144
Peach	1 unit (150g)	63
Tangerine	1 unit (100g)	50
National white grape	1 small bunch	130
Pass grape	1 tablespoon (18g)	54
Milk		
Milk cream	1 tablespoon (15g)	37
Milk with chocolate	1 cup (200ml)	222
Condensed milk	1 tablespoon (20g)	65
Buffalo milk	1 cup (240ml)	253
Goat milk	1 cup (240ml)	220
Soy milk	1 cup (240ml)	120
Skim powdered milk	2 tablespoons (40g)	73

Whole milk powder	1 tablespoon (20g)	99
Whole milk	1 cup (240ml)	150
Long-life milk with iron	1 cup (240ml)	146
Semi-skimmed milk	1 cup (240ml)	115
Eggs		
Omelet	1 serving (100g)	170
Quail egg	1 unit	33
Boiled chicken egg	1 unit	78
Fried chicken egg	1 unit	108
Scrambled egg	1 serving (100g)	195
Vegetables, greens, and grains		
Pumpkin	1 serving (100g)	40
Cress	1 serving (100g)	28
Fried Cassava	1 tea saucer (100g)	353
Lettuce	2 sheets (20g)	4
Peanut	1 serving (100g)	549
Cooked white rice	1 tablespoon (25g)	41
Cooked brown rice	1 tablespoon (20g)	22
Cooked asparagus	2 stalks (20g)	4
Black olive	1 unit (3g)	4
Green olive	1 unit (4g)	5

Roasted sweet potatoes	1 unit (100g)	143
Sweet Potato Fries	1 unit (100g)	383
French fries	1 serving (70g)	220
Aubergine	1 unit (250g)	489
Beetroot	1 small (125g)	55
Broccoli	1 tea saucer (80g)	23
Onion	1 unit (70g)	32
Cooked onion	1 unit (100g)	54
Carrot	1 unit (100g)	45
Cooked carrot	1 unit (100g)	54
Cooked cauliflower	1 serving (100g)	41
Pickled peas	1 tablespoon (20g)	19
Escarole	2 sheets (20g)	7
Spinach	1 tea saucer (100g)	38
Cooked white beans	1 tablespoon (20g)	24
Cooked and dehydrated beans	1 tablespoon (20g)	78
Cooked black beans	1 tablespoon (20g)	14
Fried manioc	1 tea saucer (100g)	352
Raw palm heart	1 tea saucer (100g)	26

Canned heart of palm	1 unit (100g)	22
Raw cucumber with peel	1 unit (150g)	21
Unpeeled raw cucumber	1 unit (150g)	5
Cabbage	1 serving (100g)	33
Cooked cabbage	1 serving (100g)	13
Cooked tomato	1 unit (100g)	18
Ripe tomato	1 unit (100g)	20
Cooked green beans	1 serving (100g)	52
Bread		
Cornbread	1 unit	150
Croissant	1 unit (60g)	247
English potato bread	1 unit (30g)	90
Wholegrain rye bread	1 slice	58
French bread	1 unit (50g)	135
A traditional loaf of bread	1 slice	74
Hamburger bread	1 unit (100g)	278
Hot-dog bread	1 unit (100g)	286
Honey bread with chocolate icing	1 unit (20g)	91
Cheese bread	1 unit (20g)	68
Whole wheat bread	1 slice (100g)	261

Whole pita bread	1 unit (50g)	147
Rolled oats	1 tablespoon (15g)	50
corn flakes	1 plate (110g)	217
Peanut Flour	1 tablespoon (15g)	56
Rice flour	1 tablespoon (15g)	53
Raw oatmeal	1 tablespoon (15g)	57
Sweet potato flour	1 tablespoon (15g)	52
English potato flour	1 tablespoon (15g)	53
Cornmeal flour	1 tablespoon (20g)	69
Cassava flour	1 tablespoon (15g)	54
Whole cornflour	1 tablespoon (15g)	30
Breadcrumbs	1 tablespoon (15g)	54
Wheat flour	1 tablespoon (15g)	54
Granola with chestnuts	1 cup of tea (60g)	300
Raw oat grain	1 tablespoon (15g)	48
Wheat germ	1 tablespoon	55

	(15g)	
Maisena	1 tablespoon (15g)	52
Powdered malt	1 tablespoon (15g)	56
Homemade dishes and processed products		
Rice and beans	2 tablespoons (40g)	75
Steak with parmigiana	1 steak	485
Pot Meat	1 steak (100g)	230
Corn cream with milk and cornstarch	1 tablespoon (20g)	72
Chicken pie	1 slice (100g)	359
Chess Chicken	1 serving	180
Fish stew	1 shell	325
Pancake	1 unit (30g)	60
Roasted pepper with meat	1 unit (200g)	298
Oxtail	1 serving	389
Ratatoille	1 tablespoon (20g)	38
Potato salad	1 cup of tea (100g)	147
Shrimp pie	1 slice (100g)	310
Sandwiches		
Hot dog with	1 unit	624

mayonnaise and vinaigrette sauce		
Hot dog with ketchup	1 unit	314
Hot dog with mustard	1 unit	330
Hot dog with ketchup and mustard	1 unit	342
Cheeseburger	1 unit	305
Cheese salad with mayonnaise	1 unit	738
Hamburger	1 unit	296
Grilled ham and cheese	1 unit	283
Sausage sandwich	1 unit	370
Turkey breast sandwich	1 unit	220
Hot cheese sandwich	1 unit	340
Tuna salad sandwich	1 unit	417

Chapter Three

Weight Loss

Quality of life is a worldwide concern, and healthy eating together with regular physical activity is essential to achieve it. Regular exercise has numerous health benefits: it improves cardiorespiratory fitness, reduces stress and the risk of diseases such as diabetes and hypertension, in addition to increasing energy expenditure and improving mood and motor coordination.

However, it is necessary to combine physical activity with a balanced diet, to prepare the body for the effort, providing the necessary nutrients that vary with the type of exercise performed and the objective that is to be achieved, such as weight loss or muscle mass gain (discussed in the next chapter).

The energy needs change with exercise, as they lead to physiological and biochemical adaptations that determine greater nutritional needs. The dietary prescription should be based on the calculation of metabolism, thus offering not only the ideal caloric amount but also carbohydrates and proteins to guarantee energy production and muscle recovery.

Demystifying Weight loss

Losing weight is a physiological process that consists of loss of body mass and weight loss, as the main consequence of the loss of reserve adipose tissue. Weight loss depends essentially on the following factors:

- Acceleration of metabolism: for the body to consume more energy than what is introduced through food;

- A low-calorie diet: for the introduction of energy into the body to be less than that spent by the body;

- Impact of diet on increasing metabolism: some foods rich in protein can accelerate metabolism;

The balance between a low-calorie diet and an increase in metabolism is the perfect duo for a healthy weight loss plan.

Generally, when we intend to lose weight our body must work essentially based on catabolic processes, which are characterized by the degradation of energy reserve tissues. However, catabolism is not a selective process: when we start a diet aimed at losing weight, in addition to losing reserve tissues, we can also lose other tissues, such as muscles. For this reason, it is always necessary to follow a weight loss diet carefully and judiciously, under the supervision of a health professional.

How to speed up metabolism

For many, the secret to losing weight quickly is, of course, to speed up your metabolism, without having to decrease your calorie intake significantly. Our metabolism is the set of reactions and biochemical processes that take place in our body to produce energy from food and thus supply it to cells.

To speed up metabolism, it is necessary to increase the energy expenditure of our body. This process depends on 3 factors:

- Basal metabolism

- Thermogenesis resulting from feeding

- Physical activity

The basal metabolic rate is the minimum energy expenditure necessary to keep vital functions functioning, which represents up to 70% of the total energy we consume. Up to 30% of energy expenditure is dependent on physical activity, while 10 to 15% depends on food digestion.

To speed up metabolism, it is necessary to increase lean mass, that is, muscle mass, and to intensify physical activity, responsible for toning the muscles.

Is it possible to lose weight without starving?

To lose weight quickly and healthily, it is imperative to eat well. As we analyzed, following only a low-calorie diet is harmful and generates muscle mass losses, a condition that consequently results in the deceleration of basal metabolism and, thus, in the easy recovery of the kilograms previously lost.

A diet that aims to lose weight must respect the needs of our body, with emphasis on its nutrition. It is possible to lose weight by eating and it is imperative to eat to lose weight. It is important, yes, to follow a balanced and healthy diet, introducing all the nutrients that our body needs.

How to lose weight? The rules for doing it healthily

The only effective way to lose weight is to follow a healthy diet and lifestyle. Trying to lose weight as quickly as possible without taking into account all the factors involved in the functioning of our body can be dangerous and it is always useless: in a short time, more fat will be gained.

To lose weight in a healthy and thus sustainable way it is important to keep the following rules in mind:

- Measure conditions at the beginning (basal metabolism, age, type and level of physical activity, diet, health conditions) to customize and adjust the weight loss process for each individual;

- Control hydration;

- Practice regular and continuous physical activity to increase lean mass;

- Balancing and adjusting the diet to meet the needs of the body, speeding up metabolism, and preventing fat accumulation.

Types of body fat

In excess, bad fats cause folds in the waist, increased circumference of the hips, legs, and arms. Also, this type of fat compromises the health and aesthetics of the body. But, be aware that not all types of body fat are harmful. Some are essential for our body.

In this book, you will learn about the 6 types of body fat and how you can fight the fat tissue considered bad. Follow!

1. Essential fat

Did you know that we need a minimum of fat in our body? That's because fat works to balance body temperature, absorb vitamins and produce various hormones.

Also, it functions as the main component of the cell membrane, along with proteins.

In this way, essential fat acts as an energy reserve for various organs such as the lungs, heart, liver, and brain.

2. White fat

This is bad fat, the one that insists on staying even if you maintain a balanced diet and practice physical exercises.

It has this name because it is white due to its low amount of blood vessels.

White fat corresponds to 90% of the body's adipose tissue. Its main function is to protect our organs in situations of falls and other accidents.

The bad news is that, in excess in the body, it causes a series of health problems.

This type of fat is the main reserve of triglycerides in our body, and responsible for promoting resistance to leptin, a hormone responsible for satiety.

That is, a person with a lot of leptin in the body tends to feel more hungry, eat more food, and put on weight.

3. Brown fat

Brown fat is a good adipose tissue, and its main function is to insulate the body. It works unlike white fat, which burns calories to fulfill its role.

It is brown because many blood vessels pass through it. This type of fat is also responsible for regulating our body temperature, but the amount of this adipose tissue is not very high in our body.

4. Beige fat

As with brown fat, beige fat also burns calories to produce heat and keep your body temperature in an appropriate range.

This type of fat comes from white fat. It changes color to beige when we exercise.

Beige fat contributes to the transformation of white (bad) to brown (good) fat.

Thus, the practice of physical activities not only helps to burn harmful fat but also favors the production of good fat.

5. Visceral fat

This is the most harmful type of fat of all, and it consists of white fat that is deposited between the organs, mainly in the abdomen.

It is also quite visible in the peritoneal cavity, a region that lies between the abdomen and the pelvis.

The excess accumulation of this type of fat is related to a greater propensity to various diseases, such as hypertension.

Another harm is that it decreases metabolism, and consequently the burning of fat, in addition to aggravating inflammatory processes.

6. Subcutaneous fat

This is the type of fat that makes it impossible to see the muscles. It is just under the skin and is easier to perceive.

It is not as harmful as white or visceral fat, but it is responsible for making the appearance of the body more round. Also, this is the fat responsible for the appearance of cellulite.

How to avoid body fat types

To avoid all types of bad fats, those that are bad for our body, it is best to maintain a balanced diet and exercise regularly.

Body mass index

Nutrition plays an important role in maintaining health. If a person does not eat properly from a medical point of view, he may develop several different diseases, such as pancreatitis, cholecystitis, cholelithiasis, atherosclerosis, coronary heart disease, stroke, diabetes mellitus, disorders of the musculoskeletal system, some cancers, etc.

A healthy diet must meet the body's needs for energy, nutrients, and maintain a healthy weight, fitness, and vitality.

BODY MASS INDEX (BMI) is a simple ratio of weight for height, often used to classify obesity and overweight. The index is calculated as the ratio of body weight in kilograms to the square of height in meters (kg / m^2). BMI is the most convenient measure of obesity and overweight in a population since it is the same for both sexes and all age groups of adults.

Body mass index is calculated using the formula:

$$I = \frac{m}{h^2},$$

Where

- m is the mass of a person in kilograms
- h - person's height in meters

For example, your height is 1.7 m, your body weight is 78 kg. We square 1.7 m - we get 2.89 m^2. After that, we divide 78 kg by 2.89 m^2. We get a figure of 26.9, which will be your BMI, indicating that you are overweight.

Interpreting BMI indicators

According to the recommendations of the World Health Organization (WHO), your BMI result should be interpreted as follows:

Indicator	Body mass index (kg/m^2)
Norm	less than 25
Overweight	25-29.9
I degree of obesity	30-34.9
II degree obesity	35-39.9
III degree of obesity	more than 40

Relationship between body mass index (BMI) and disease risk

BMI	Health risk
Less than 18.5 kg / m^2	Reduced weight. You need to eat better
18.5-24.9 kg / m^2	Normal body weight, no cause for concern
25.0-29.9 kg / m^2	Overweight and the risk of developing atherosclerosis, diabetes, and other diseases
30.0-39.9 kg / m^2	Severely overweight (obese), increased health risk
More than 40 kg / m^2	Severely overweight (overweight). The health risk is very high.

There is also a simpler method for determining the risk of developing atherosclerosis, diabetes mellitus, and other diseases.

Health implications of excess body fat

Being overweight and obese is the result of the formation of abnormal or excessive body fat that can be harmful to health.

Body mass index (BMI) is a simple ratio of body weight for height, often used to diagnose obesity and overweight in adults. The index is calculated as the ratio of body weight in kilograms to the square of height in meters (kg/m^2).

What causes overweight and obesity?

The main cause of obesity and overweight is an energy imbalance, in which the caloric content of the diet exceeds the energy requirements of the body. The following trends are noted throughout the world:

- increased consumption of foods with high energy density and high-fat content;
- decreased physical activity due to the increasingly sedentary nature of many activities, changes in travel patterns, and increasing urbanization.

What are the most common health effects of being overweight and obese?

An elevated BMI is one of the main risk factors for non-communicable diseases such as:

- cardiovascular disease (mainly heart disease and stroke), which was the leading cause of death in 2012;
- diabetes;
- disorders of the musculoskeletal system (especially osteoarthritis - an extremely disabling degenerative joint disease);

- some oncological diseases (including cancer of the endometrium, breast, ovary, prostate, liver, gallbladder, kidney, and colon).

The risk of these non-communicable diseases increases as BMI increases.

How can the problem of overweight and obesity be reduced?

Overweight and obesity, as well as related noncommunicable diseases, are largely preventable. Incentive environments and community-based support are critical for people to make decisions about healthier diets and regular physical activity as the most appropriate choice (that is, affordable and feasible) to help prevent overweight and obesity ...

On an individual level, everyone can:

- limit the calorie content of your diet by reducing the amount of consumed fats and sugars;
- increase your intake of fruits and vegetables, as well as pulses, whole grains, and nuts;
- engage in regular physical activity (60 minutes a day for children and 150 minutes a week for adults).

Fat burning tips

There are two types of fat in our body - subcutaneous and internal. The subcutaneous "only" spoil the reflection in the mirror, while the really dangerous one is the inner one. It accumulates around the organs and interferes with their normal functioning.

To lose weight through subcutaneous fat, rather than water and muscle, you need to eat and exercise properly. It is important to understand that fat burning is a long-term process that requires discipline and consistency. And no matter how much we want to lose weight quickly, we will not be able to deceive the body, and harm ourselves. So let's burn subcutaneous fat in the mind!

1. A 100-meter sprint run 10 times will save you 500 calories.

2. Put on a sweatshirt before training - a heated body loses calories faster.

3. Power yoga burns 344 calories in one session.

4. One workout per week can be done on an empty stomach. This will keep your adrenaline levels high and your blood sugar low.

5. Interval running is very effective for weight loss.

6. If you attend classes with your loved one, the likelihood of continuing training for a long time increases.

7. A visit to the pool is also useful in losing weight. And especially running in the water (you need to get your feet to the bottom).

8. When exercising on elliptical trainers, be sure to use your arms. Due to this, the muscles of the arms will be worked out, and calories will be burned faster.

9. The training program should be changed in 4-6 months.

10. When exercising on the treadmill, focus on hard work, do not look at the screen.

11. When doing squats, use a lot of weight. In this case, more muscles will be involved.

12. It is also recommended to swing the press with a large weight.

13. It is very useful to combine cardio and strength training. Jump rope between sets, or incorporate some exercise into your circuit workout.

14. Get up off the couch at last - during commercials, do some push-ups, squats, and jumps. This is a great light workout for burning fat.

15. A ten-minute skipping rope session is equivalent to the number of calories burned from a fifteen-minute run.

16. After a tough workout, eat a slice of whole-grain bread with peanut butter to avoid overeating.

17. Make burpees. This compound exercise trains virtually every muscle.

18. Push-ups every morning will give you energy for the whole day and strengthen your upper body.

19. Resistance jogging is a great way to lose weight. Working with an elastic band will make running harder and burn more calories.

20. After every 800 km buy yourself a new trainer, this will increase your motivation and, therefore, the result!

21. You can also use a pedometer. It will be great if you walk 10 thousand steps a day.

22. Working with complex equipment (e.g. sandbags or tires) will have the added benefit of increasing mass and strength.

23. Working out with a stronger friend will give you extra motivation.

24. The training mix of different martial arts is very original. This can include plyometric and supersets, reducing rest time.

25. Don't forget about pull-ups

26. It is very important to keep your parameters under control - the number of calories, body weight, percentage of body fat, etc.

27. While waiting in line for the treadmill, you can do a few sets of box jumps or climbing climbers to warm up.

28. When doing strength exercises, it is necessary to reduce the rest time by 2 times.

29. Training should include both strength training and cardio.

30. If you have to skip a workout, you can work out with an elastic band at home (also on free days from classes).

31. Fractional nutrition (6 times a day in small portions) speeds up metabolism. You need to eat every 3-4 hours.

32. Keep 20 minutes between the first and second courses.

33. Use smaller plates.

34. The blue color reduces appetite. You can use blue dishes.

35. Mayonnaise and sour cream are excellent substitutes for homemade yogurt, which helps to get rid of 700 and 100 calories in ½ cup.

36. By peeling nuts, you will eat 2 times less.

37. After eating, you can chew sugar-free mint gum. Peppermint signals the brain to stop eating.

38. For a snack, you can use a few pistachios instead of a sandwich.

39. For tomorrow, it is better to eat oatmeal and eggs saturated with protein.

40. Eat in the kitchen, not on the couch.

41. It is important to drink plenty of water. People often confuse the desire to drink with hunger.

42. Eggs, poultry, and fish are best eaten boiled rather than fried.

43. Add skim milk to coffee instead of cream and sugar, which will eliminate the additional 105 calories.

44. When cooking meat and fish, roll them in bread crumbs, not eggs and flour. This will reduce calories. Cook the chicken without the skin.

45. Fiber-rich strawberries are a great addition to a protein shake.

46. Avocados are full of essential fats.

47. The number of potatoes and pasta per week should be no more than a soccer ball.

48. In restaurants, choose steamed dishes.

49. Tea is very rich in antioxidants that burn fat.

50. The maximum amount of sugar per day should be 72 g.

51. Popcorn instead of chips for a snack saves 60 kcal.

52. Legumes are packed with fiber and protein and help fight obesity.

53. Plan every meal carefully. If you've been sticking to the program all week and then suddenly gorged up, it will nullify all efforts.

54. In a cafe, prefer chicken sticks to chicken wings. They are cooked without skin, which means they contain more protein and much less fat, salt, and calories.

55. It is necessary to give up the usual dishes gradually - this reduces the likelihood of a breakdown.

56. When preparing food, taste it from the opposite end of the spoon. This will allow you to consume much fewer calories.

57. Eat more foods that contain fiber.

58. Replace milk chocolate with black. It contains less sugar and more energy-boosting antioxidants.

59. When preparing a salad, season it with balsamic vinegar, it is less high in calories.

60. If you give up burgers, you will not gain an extra 300 kcal.

61. Keep a record of everything you eat. Then reduce the volume by 250 kcal per day, and you can lose 1 kg per month.

62. Don't skip breakfast. A nutrient-rich breakfast is, oddly enough, a great way to lose weight. Eat a healthy breakfast of 400-600 calories within an hour of waking up.

63. Outside the house, make ½ portion and wrap the rest with you.

64. Get rid of temptations - do not leave candy, etc. in a conspicuous place.

65. Throwing a party? Bring leftover chips, cookies, and cake to work rather than leaving them at home. Let the employees finish everything for you.

66. For dessert, you can eat low-fat chocolate, it is much less high in calories.

67. Don't order home delivery. Cook at home and you will always know what you are eating.

68. Replace the cooking oil with a special oil spray. One spray only contains 10 calories and 1 g of fat (versus 102 cal and 12 g).

69. Buy only one serving of your favorite snack. It's better to order a second portion later than to force yourself to finish it out of greed.

70. Use spices. Fiery spices (and hot peppers) boost metabolism. Besides, using such spices you will not be able to eat very quickly.

71. One tablespoon of oil contains about 100 calories. You can reduce the amount by mixing equal parts of peanut butter with boiled carrots or sweet potatoes.

72. Avoid processed foods containing industrial and trans fats. After all, trans fats can be very harmful to your health and will not allow you to lose weight.

73. A serving of macaroni and cheese can be substituted for a half cup of cauliflower and pumpkin puree with ½ cup of grated cheese.

74. Chew slowly.

75. Turkey is much less high in calories than beef.

76. Eat rice with broccoli and other low-calorie vegetables.

77. In a cafe, ask for the sauce separately. This will help you eat a smaller portion.

78. Products are often labeled "0 kcal", but you should be aware that manufacturers label all products that contain no more than 5 kcal.

79. Eat low-fat cottage cheese.

80. From alcohol, give preference to light beer or a glass of wine. Don't drink mixed drinks.

81. Throw out all unnecessary things from the kitchen. By letting go of temptation, you are more likely to stick to the plan.

82. Go in for rock climbing.

83. Take your photo "before".

84. Ride your bike to work.

85. Use a variety of fitness programs for your phone (Fast Food, Calorie Counter, or Electronic Workout Diary). Or ask a friend to write you motivational messages.

86. Find your limit. You have understood that it is time to change. When did it happen? Start from this moment.

87. Daily walks with the dog for 20 minutes will help you lose 6 kg in a year.

88. Write short-term goals on cards. Once you get it done, add it to your heap. Visual achievements will increase self-confidence.

89. Get a physical examination. Poor health and infrequent visits to the doctor reduce the chances of success and do not promote weight loss.

90. Don't ride elevators. 10 minutes of climbing the stairs save you 100 calories.

91. Before you start cleaning the aftermath of the party, eat a few fruits, then there will be no desire to snack on chips or cookies.

92. Playing basketball will save you 500 calories.

93. You need to sleep at least 7 hours a day. Not getting enough sleep slows down your metabolism.

94. Stress triggers the release of the hormone cortisol, which increases appetite.

95. Take the kids to the park. You can practice there while the children are walking.

96. Run. Increase the time by 1 minute every day.

97. Do your household chores. Ironing burns 166 calories per hour, washing floors and making bed 149 calories.

98. Go shirtless. You will see your accomplishments in the mirror and it will give you motivation.

99. Take 30 minutes of exercise every day. Don't eat fast food.

100. Do crosswords while watching TV. You will think less about food when your hands are full.

Maybe you still think that losing weight is too difficult. Perhaps this is true for some, but not for you. After all, just by reading this book, you have already lost 60 to 100 calories. You are the master of your life. And by adding the weight loss exercises to it, you will achieve an amazing result!

Exercises to aid fat burning

Every girl dreams of losing weight and getting rid of fat in the thighs, buttocks, and abdomen. After all, it is in these places that fat quickly accumulates, and getting rid of it is not so easy! And these are the most difficult places in the struggle for harmony and fit. But that doesn't mean giving up! For slender legs and a flat tummy, you just need to train regularly! They will help you look beautiful and fit.

You need to do a set of exercises, which we will discuss below, 3 times a week for 40 minutes. Of course, it all depends on your determination and problem areas.

The benefits of these exercises are that they not only help you lose fat, but they also help to improve muscle tone throughout the body!

To speed up the process of losing weight, you must also increase activity. Be active during the day, take walks in the evening. If you are planning a vacation, then do something active, play tennis, ride a bike, and the like.

Fat Burning Workout Plan

- First, start your workout with warm-up and cardio.

- And the last is the bar (1 to 5 minutes). Increase the time each time.

- All exercises are performed 30 sec. activity/30 sec. recreation.

1. Running with high knees

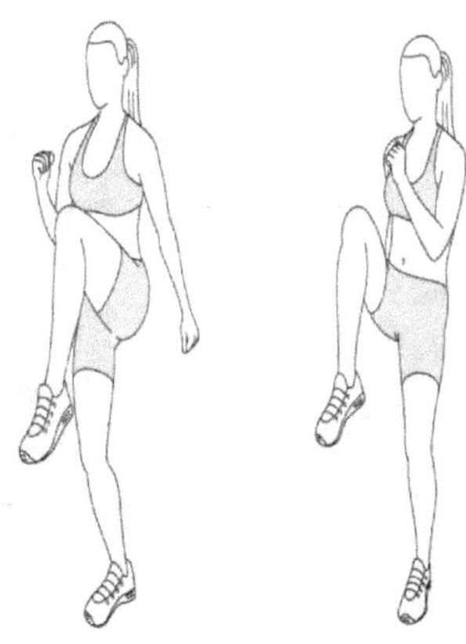

Execution technique:

In the starting position, take a pose with bent knees, put your feet shoulder-width apart. Timed 30 seconds and run in place, lifting your knees as high as possible to your stomach. You need to run as fast as you can. After 30 seconds of running, rest for 20-30 seconds.

2. Jumping with arms and legs

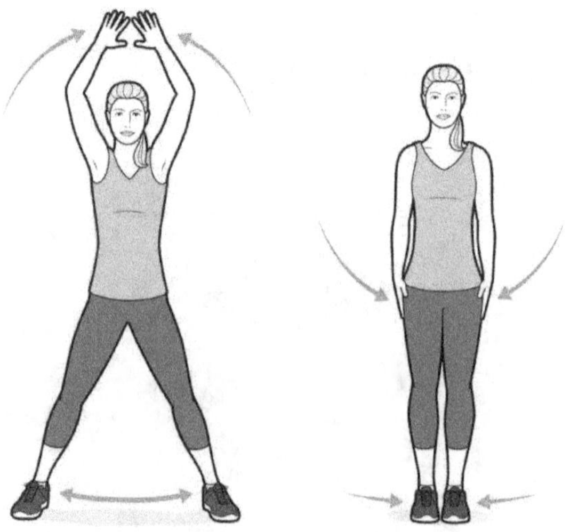

Execution technique:

First, you need to stand up straight, keep your arms and legs together. Then breathe in and jump upward with it, spreading your arms and legs at the same time. When you return to the opposite position, exhale. These jumps need to be done 30 after that rest for 20-30 seconds.

3. Burpees

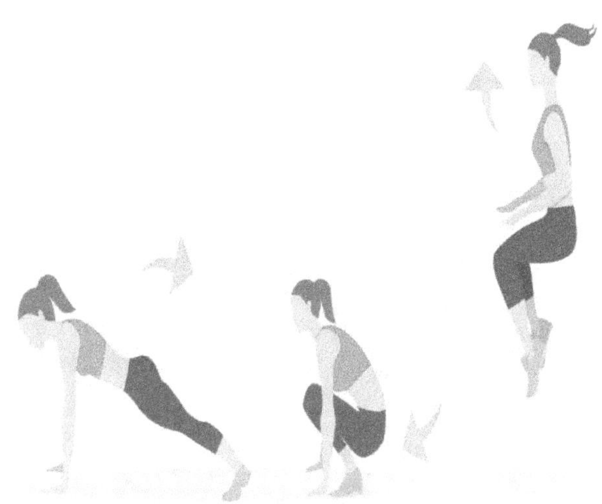

This exercise is considered one of the most effective for burning fat. Besides, during work, the maximum number of muscles are involved: arms, chest, quadriceps, gluteal muscles, biceps, hips, and abs. By doing them, you can also become more resilient and develop coordination.

Execution technique:

Starting position - you need to sit down and put your hands on the floor. Then make an emphasis while lying, return to the squat position and jump up from this position. Do this exercise 10 times, and after completing it, rest for 30 seconds.

4. Bodyweight squats

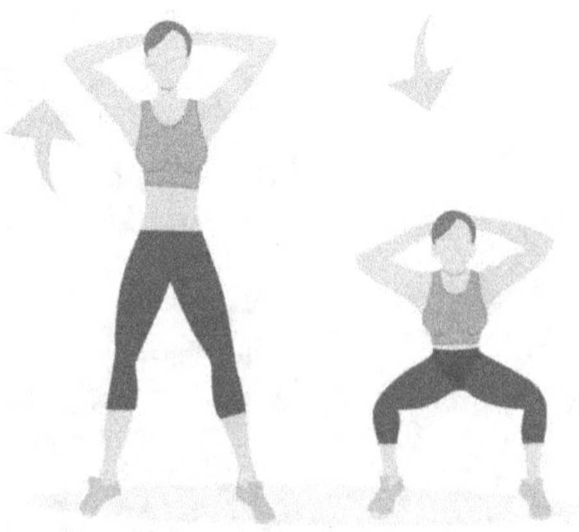

Execution technique:

Start by placing your hands behind your head or in front of you. Then place your feet shoulder-width apart. As you go down, you need to tighten your abs and buttocks. Go down as you exhale, and as you inhale, rise. Repeat the exercise 12 times in 3 sets. Rest 30 seconds between sets.

5. Twisting with the ball

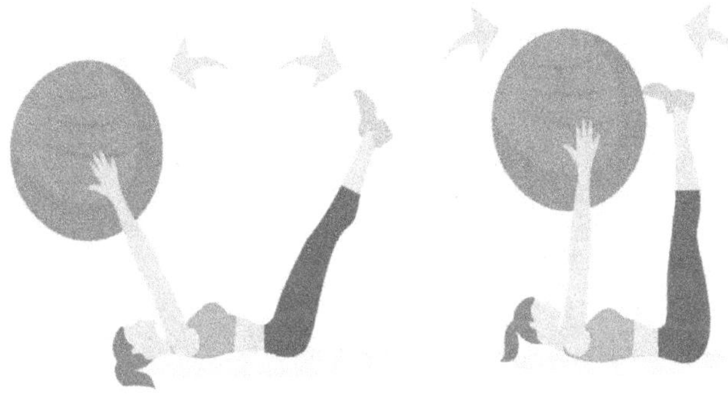

This exercise works well on the lower abdomen. A ball is needed to complete it. Not necessarily just a fitball, if you don't have one, then you can use the usual or other means at hand.

Execution technique:

Lie on the floor in an equal position. Place the ball in your hands. Hands should be equal. Then you need to simultaneously raise your legs and arms with the ball and make them meet in the middle. Then turn them in the opposite position, just do not touch the floor. Watch your breath as you do it. While lifting your legs and arms, inhale and when lowering, exhale. You need to do the exercise 12 times in 3 sets.

6. Swing one leg

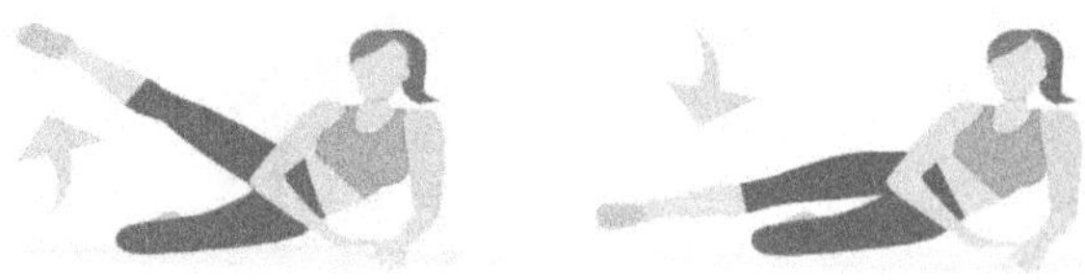

With this exercise, you can work out the muscles of the buttocks and lateral press well.

Execution technique:

First, you need to lie on the floor, you can use a special rug. Then rest on your hand and raise your torso a little. The leg you are lying on must be bent. You need to lift your free leg, and you should not completely lower it onto the lower leg. Make sure your foot is straight. When you raise it, you need to inhale, and as you exhale, lower it. Do 10 lifts on one leg and 10 lifts on the second, 3 sets each. Rest 30 seconds between sets.

You can add a fitness elastic to this exercise in the future. With its help, you can slightly complicate the load and better work out the muscles of the hips and buttocks!

7. Exercise "*Bridge*"

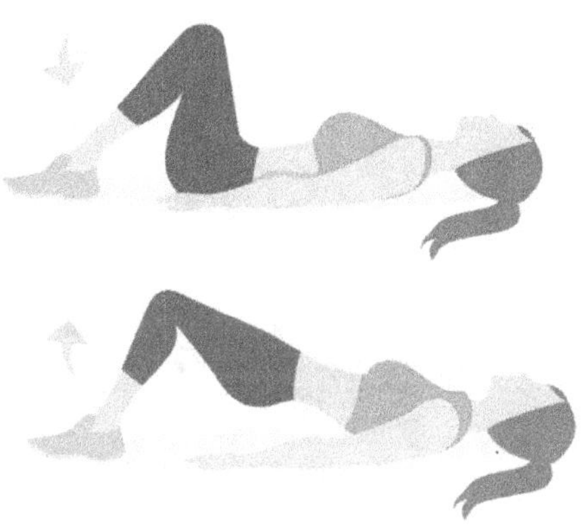

This exercise is good for the hips and pelvis, and it also promotes muscle development in the legs.

Execution technique:

First, you need to lie down on the floor. At this point, bend your legs and your feet should be on the floor. Keep your arms straight, palms down. You need to lift the pelvis so that one straight line forms from the knees to the head. At this time, the buttocks should be tense. When lifting, inhale, and when you lower your pelvis, exhale. The exercise must be done 10 times in 3 sets. You can rest for 30 seconds between sets.

After doing the exercise often, it may seem light, then you can complicate it a little by adding a little weight or straightening one leg and raising the pelvis along with the equal leg

8. Elbow plank

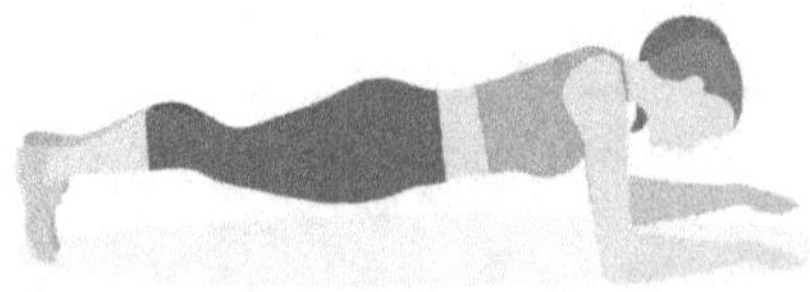

It is always good to do the plank as a finishing exercise. This will solidify your results. As you know, the plank engages almost all muscle groups, so you can strengthen your muscles, abdomen, waist, legs, back, neck, and shoulders.

Execution technique:

At the very beginning, you need to lie down on the floor. Place your elbows on the floor in front of you and focus on them. Don't raise your head. Keep your gaze down. As for the legs, keep them equal too. When you get into the bar, then you should keep your whole body in tension. All parts must form one solid line. When you get into the plank, start with 30 seconds. Then lower yourself to the floor. Repeat the exercise 3 times. When you feel like you can stand for more, increase the time to 1-2 minutes.

Bravo!

Must-Have Tips to Remember

Pay attention to nutrition

Performing the set of exercises above, do not forget about nutrition. After all, this is 50% of all success! Review your entire diet. Exclude from it all harmful, flour, sweet. Forget about fast food and quick bites with sausage sandwiches.

- Your food should be low in calories, and your meals should contain as many fruits, vegetables, and proteins as possible. Try to refuse any sauces, because they greatly increase the calorie content of dishes.

- As for drinks, you should give up soda and drink as much plain clean water as possible. According to statistics, a person should drink 2 liters a day. If you want something hot, then drink tea without sugar, and choose coffee without caffeine.

Reduce stress

Stress causes the body to release the hormone cortisol. Cortisol affects metabolism and stimulates the cravings for sugar and other refined carbohydrates. This causes fat to build up in our bodies.

Train your cortisol level and your extra weight will be done.

People who experience high levels of stress are more likely to experience fatigue. In this case, it may seem attractive to order fast food instead of preparing healthy meals at home.

It could also mean they are exercising less. All of these habits can quickly lead to weight gain.

How to reduce stress levels? The following tips can help with this:

- Exercise, do regular exercise, even if it's a daily walk

- Eat a balanced diet

- Try meditation

- Take deep breaths

- Spend time in nature

If you perform the above exercises and recommendations in good faith, then you will be able to achieve results and you can forget about your shortcomings!

Consistency is the key to achieving your cherished goal. Maintain an exercise regimen that combines aerobic exercise and strength training for the best results. The main thing is to believe in yourself and then everything will work out for you!

30 days diet plan

Here are some sample diet choices that you can use to create your own personalized 30 days meal plan for weight loss.

Breakfast	First snack	Lunch	Second snack	Dinner
Oatmeal and some dried fruit, low-fat milk, and fruit.	Fruits or crackers with feta cheese.	Chicken and vegetable soup. Chopped tomatoes, cucumbers, bell peppers, onions, and lettuce with olive oil.	One glass of curdled milk (2.5% fat) and two-grain loaves.	Baked bell pepper stuffed with brown rice and minced beef. Cherry tomatoes with soft cheese and some herbs.
Vegetable	Low-fat	Broccoli	Oatmeal	Fish fillet

salad with olive oil. Hot whole-grain sandwich.	cottage cheese, fresh or frozen berries.	baked with cod. Fresh lettuce leaf.	cookies, green tea.	with vegetables. Natural yogurt.
Oatmeal porridge with a spoonful of raisins.	One glass of kefir (1% fat) and two-grain loaves.	Boiled, stewed, or baked skinless chicken breast with boiled rice. Light vegetable salad.	Natural yogurt (1.5% fat), diet bread.	Grilled or braised lean fish. Greens salad dressed with lemon juice.
Boiled buckwheat with a tablespoon of vegetable	One apple, low-fat cottage cheese.	Veal with steamed potatoes. Tomato and feta cheese	Low-fat cottage cheese with honey.	Salmon with rice garnish. Tomato slicing.

oil.		salad.		
Scrambled eggs, a large tomato, cheese, and black bread sandwich.	Fruits or crackers with feta cheese.	Vegetarian soup with a slice of second-rate bread. Vegetable salad dressed with olive oil.	Low-calorie yogurt, some oatmeal cookies.	Two-protein omelet with low-fat milk, tomato, and green onions.
Low fat cottage cheese mixed with parsley, radish, and herbs.	Low-fat cheese and diet bread.	Grilled lean fish and boiled potatoes. Herbs salad dressed with lemon juice.	Boiled egg, tomato.	Casserole with cheese, lean veal, and vegetables. A sandwich made from second-rate bread

				and pink salmon.
Buckwheat with boiled chicken, lettuce.	One boiled egg and a glass of vegetable juice.	Stewed liver with buckwheat garnish. Vegetable mix.	Kefir with black bread.	Stewed or baked veal. Fresh cabbage salad.

By following all the rules and exercises, you can achieve the desired result in 30 days.

Good luck!

Chapter Four

Muscle Gain

Muscle gain for male

Resistance training is a process of exercising with external resistance to improve skeletal muscle performance, appearance, or a combination of the two. Resistance training can simultaneously increase muscle strength and size, however, there is a clear distinction between training the ability to produce a maximum effort and targeting muscle growth. By itself, resistance training does not cause muscle growth; fatigue-inducing exercise stress stimulates the physiological mechanisms responsible for increasing muscle mass.

According to the principle of overloading when building an exercise program, to stimulate physiological changes, such as muscle growth, it is necessary to apply physical stimuli at a greater intensity than the body is habitually receiving. Muscle growth from resistance training occurs as a result of an increase in muscle fiber thickness and fluid volume in the sarcoplasm of muscle cells. Understanding how the muscular system adapts to the effects of resistance training can help you determine the best training method to maximize muscle growth in your clients. Existing research explains to us how the body can respond to stimuli, but each person can get slightly different results in response to the effects of resistance exercise.

The ability to gain muscle mass and increase lean muscle mass depends on a variety of variables, including gender, age, experience with resistance training, genetics, sleep, nutrition, and fluid intake. Emotional and physical stressors, each of which can affect the adaptation of physiological systems to resistance training, can also affect the ability to increase mass. For example, overworking at work or not getting enough sleep can dramatically decrease muscle growth. Knowing the correct application of this science, however, can have a significant impact in empowering you to help clients achieve maximum results.

How to gain muscle growth

On screens and in magazines, we see beautiful relief bodies, there are so many of them in the media, and so few in life. Everyone mentally "tries on" these images, but few get down to business. But reaching the perfect body is not so difficult with the proper discipline and knowledge.

The correct strategy for gaining muscle mass is based on three pillars. If you ignore at least one of them, you can say goodbye to dreams of the body of an ancient Greek god. So, what kind of whales are we talking about?

- **FOOD**

As with losing weight, it all starts with nutrition. Nothing comes from nowhere. The body cannot just start building muscle mass even with intense strength training. Remember the words that to sell something unnecessary, you must first buy something unnecessary? So it is here. To build muscle mass, which the body has previously done without, you need to start consuming more energy than it needed before setting this goal. How do I consume more energy? That's right, with food. We read the step-by-step instructions "How to eat to gain muscle mass" and from today we are introducing these steps into our life.

Step # 1. The most boring. We count calories.

Without this, it is very difficult to know if you are eating enough and create a calorie surplus. Using the calorie count method discussed in chapter 2, we calculate our norm (taking into account how many workouts we plan per week) and increase the number of calories received by 10-20%. This is the number of calories you need to consume per day to gain muscle mass. We strongly recommend counting all calories at first, every meal. This can be stressful but will become unnecessary when the habit develops. It will be easier to count calories (and at the same time proteins, fats and carbohydrates).

Step # 2. The most difficult one. Increasing your protein intake.

Protein acts as a building block for muscles. With a lack of it, even if you eat in surplus, only fat will grow, but not muscle. You need to consume 2-2.5 g of protein per kg of body weight. That is, a person weighing 70kg needs to eat 140-175g of protein. To make sure that you are likely to have a lot less of it in your diet, add everything you eat to the supplement we mentioned above. If you realize that you cannot eat so many protein foods, but you want to gain muscle mass, protein (meaning a sports supplement) will help you. Whey protein isolate can be found at any sports store, and soy protein isolate is suitable for vegans. The protein content in them tends to 100%, the powder is diluted with water or milk and used as a cocktail.

Step # 3. Most overrated. Setting the diet

On the Internet, you can find many tips about how many meals should be, what portions, with what additives. It doesn't matter if you eat 2 times a day or 6-7. Focus on your feelings and capabilities. Choose a regimen that you can stick to REGULARLY and keep your calories and protein intake. There should be just enough meals so that you do not feel hungry. Eating a calorie intake at a time and starving all day is not a so-so option that alienates you from the result.

Step # 4. Most controversial. We plan meals before and after training.

Discussions about what to eat before and after training to gain muscle mass faster are conducted with enviable regularity, new research is constantly being carried out, new conclusions are being drawn. What to believe? Information changes all the time and will change, trying everything at once, you will only harm yourself. To get the most out of your workout, try the following guidelines:

- Do not exercise on an empty stomach, as you will only start the process of muscle destruction.

- Eating heavy meals before exercise is also harmful. You will not be able to exercise effectively, and the body will also have to spend energy digesting food.

- 40 minutes before training, drink a protein shake or eat cottage cheese, this will increase protein synthesis in the muscles and will not allow the body to destroy muscle tissue. You can also eat some fast carbs, like something sweet.

- After a workout, you can have a light snack, eating everything you want, and after a couple of hours, you should have a full meal.

Step # 5. The most commonplace. We control the consumption of fats and water.

Many odes have already been dedicated to water, we will not repeat ourselves. With regards to mass gain, the consequences of a lack of water are as follows: proteins are absorbed worse, once, muscles are not clogged with blood to failure, two. Just remember that on average, 1 kg of weight should have 25-30 ml of water. But without fanaticism, your body has a more accurate beacon than human-made rules. This beacon is thirst and follows it. Your body may have more or vice versa less than the notorious 8 glasses that everyone is talking about. Learn to hear your body and drink more pure water, rather than sugary juices and soda. As for fats, it is not only unnecessary to give them up, but also harmful: without them, the process of muscle recovery, the absorption of vitamins and protein slows down. You just need to train yourself to give preference to sources of the right fats: fish, nuts, avocados, flaxseed, and olive oil.

STRENGTH TRAINING

When you figured out how to eat to gain muscle mass, you can proceed to train. Only a coach can develop a complete training program that is right for you. This is especially important for beginners, as improper exercise technique can at best nullify all efforts, at worst - lead to injury. If you decide to practice in the gym, be sure to take at least a few classes with a coach. Here we will give only general recommendations that need to be considered when gaining muscle mass.

First, you need to understand that muscle growth can be achieved either by increasing the size of muscle fibers or by increasing their number. At first, growth is also possible by increasing blood flow and affecting the energy depot of the muscles.

Therefore, the sequence of actions will be something like this:

Start training with moderate weights in a multi-rep mode (15-20 reps per set) to provoke metabolic stress. Such training will increase the blood circulation in the muscles and maximize the branching of the vascular network. Also, training with small weights is minimally traumatic and allows you to feel the muscles and work out the technique. It is better to build a workout so that the whole body is involved. Basic exercises such as deadlifts, squats, bench presses, pull-ups are perfect. The body will "respond" with fairly rapid muscle growth, but only up to a certain limit.

After you feel that your workouts have ceased to bring results, you can begin to increase the size of muscle fibers. This process is called hypertrophy and is achieved through micro-damage to muscle fibers. The body reacts to this as if it were an injury and compensates for it with a margin during the recovery so that the injury does not recur. A very rough analogy can be drawn to skin scars. Such growth requires a constant increase in the load, that is, the weight of the training equipment. Pick a weight with which you can perform a maximum of 4-8 reps. The last rep should always be at the limit. Training days with such training are divided into muscle groups, for example, one day we train the chest, the other legs, the third back.

Since muscle cell growth is limited, progress will sooner or later stop. To achieve an increase in the number of muscle fibers, the so-called hyperplasia, volumetric high-intensity training is required. But this is a topic that requires a separate article. Moreover, before it makes sense to start this stage, it will take about two years of regular training.

Based on this, you can immediately answer the question of whether it is possible to gain muscle mass at home. You can, but only up to a certain point, since at home, you are unlikely to be able to provide a sufficient increase in the load. In any case, wherever you train, it is important to work for quality and feel the muscle that you work with.

Another axiom - the more varied your workouts, the better your growth. The body quickly enough adapts to one type of load, even small changes in exercise will provide a good shake-up. And you need to completely change the training program every 2-3 months.

• **RELAXATION**

This comes as a surprise to many, but muscle does NOT grow with exercise. The load is a kind of signal for the body to start the process of building muscle mass, while the process itself takes place exclusively at rest. Even if you want to gain muscle mass as quickly as possible, rest cannot be ignored. By not giving your muscles time to recover, you inhibit their growth. If you want to get results from training, follow these rules:

- Do not exercise for more than 2 days in a row
- The duration of the workout should not exceed 90 minutes.
- Observe the regime: sleep should last at least 7-8 hours.
- Do not exercise during illness, and afterward exercise with light weights.
- Give your body a week's rest from training every 2-3 months.

- On days of rest, it will not be superfluous to visit the bath complex, massage, take a contrast shower.
- After your workout, take at least 10-15 minutes of stretching to help relieve tension and increase muscle flexibility.

It is impossible to say how long muscles recover after training. This is an individual indicator that depends on many factors. Try to stick to 48 hours of rest between workouts, then see how it feels. If you find that you can't give your best, still feeling tired from the previous workout, try increasing the time between them. This time can be different for individual muscle groups. For example, large muscle groups can recover up to 72 hours, and most often a day is enough for the press, and you can train it at least every day.

Diet for gaining muscle mass

The golden rule for every athlete who decides to conquer the ladies with a well-built figure is to consume more than you spend. Do not be afraid that excess body fat will appear. Gaining muscle mass is a great stress for the body, and if you eat poorly, then instead of positive changes, the opposite process will occur. A metabolic disorder has not been beneficial to anyone yet, so it is important to know how many calories are needed for normal metabolism. Having learned the figure, you will understand how much you will have to consume over this measure. Calculations can be made using the following formula:

Weight (kg) x 30 = number of calories (Kcal)

In this case, as a rule, it is enough to "eat" 500 Kcal more. But do not forget about the individual characteristics of each athlete. If an ectomorph (prone to thinness) is not damaged even by 1000 Kcal, then for an endomorph (prone to overweight) more than 500 Kcal is too much, which will make itself felt by the growth of adipose tissue and not muscle. To compose a menu, it is important to know the calorie content of a particular product.

The diet should be formulated so that the average daily intake of proteins, fats, and carbohydrates is in the following proportions:

- Proteins - 20% -30%;

- Fats - 10% -20%;

- Carbohydrates - 50% -60%.

If it is difficult to remember this percentage, understand another truth: there should be little fat, protein - no more than 2 grams per 1 kg of weight, and carbohydrates - 2 times more than protein.

Exercises to build muscle

To gain muscle mass the 20-minute training plan must be carried out at least twice a week in an intense way, as it is possible to work for several muscle groups and favor the gain of muscle mass. This type of training is an interesting option for times when the person does not have much time but also does not want to stop training.

The hypertrophy training plan for those who want to gain muscle mass can be done at home, as the exercises use only the weight of the body itself, and it is not necessary to use gym equipment. This plan mixes two types of movement, the active ones, which allow a greater increase in muscle, and the isometric ones, which are perfect to help tone up.

However, to have the desired results, in addition to performing the training intensely and regularly, the person must have a healthy diet and according to the goal, being necessary to consume more calories than is spent, consume good fats and increase the amount of protein ingested during the day.

1. Barbell squats

To begin, place a barbell on the back of your shoulders at the base of your neck.

Separate your feet and hold the bar over your head, placing your hands slightly wider than shoulder-width. Pause for a second when your knees are flexed at 90 degrees and your thighs are parallel to the floor.

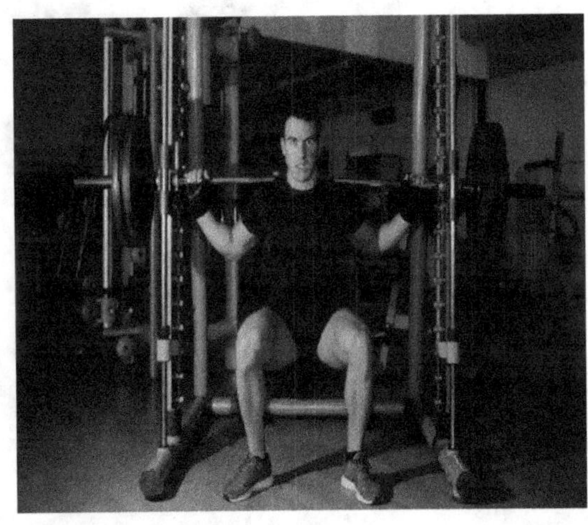

Look straight ahead, bend your knees, throw your buttocks back, slowly lower your hips to the floor and return to your starting position to complete a repetition.

Adding the resistance of a bar to challenge your limits and perform a more demanding workout will allow you to move to the next level. Therefore, we recommend that you start with just a barbell and, as you gain strength, gradually add more weight.

2. Push-ups

This is one of the best exercises for the upper body because it works everything - your chest, your back, your arms, and even your abdomen! Make sure that your shoulders are aligned with your wrists and place your elbows to the side (so as not to widen your elbows). Try to keep your chest and hips as close to the floor as possible without touching.

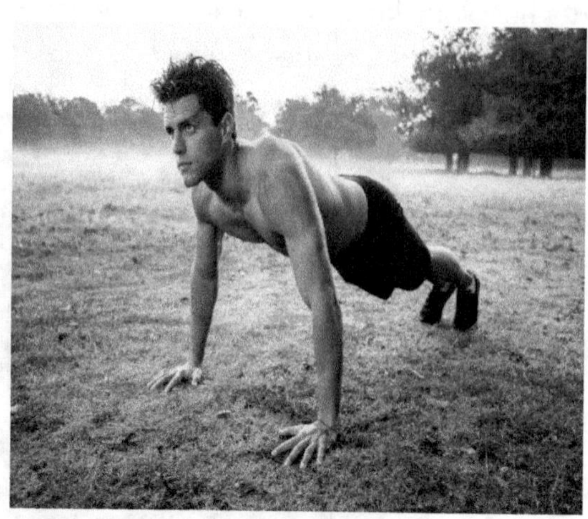

3. Advance or sink

The advance or sink works the glutes, contributing to the hardening of the butt. In addition to being one of the main exercises with the bodyweight for glutes, it also affects the posterior thigh muscles, the adductors, and the quadriceps. The exercise demands a lot from the glutes because when the hip corresponding to the front leg is well bent, the glutes are stretched and a high load is placed on top of them, right in the most difficult part of the movement.

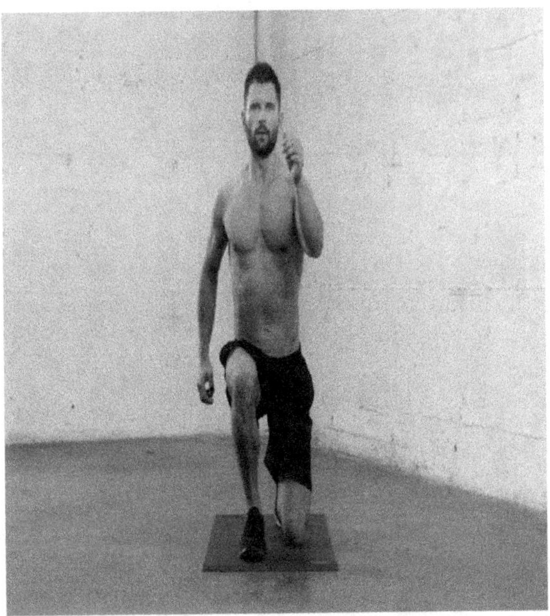

4. Board

The board has become one of the main exercises to define the central region of your body. If you are struggling to keep your arms extended and the exercise seems too tight, try to maintain the position by supporting the upper body weight on your forearms. Make sure to align your elbows and shoulders and keep your hips, heels, and shoulders at the same height.

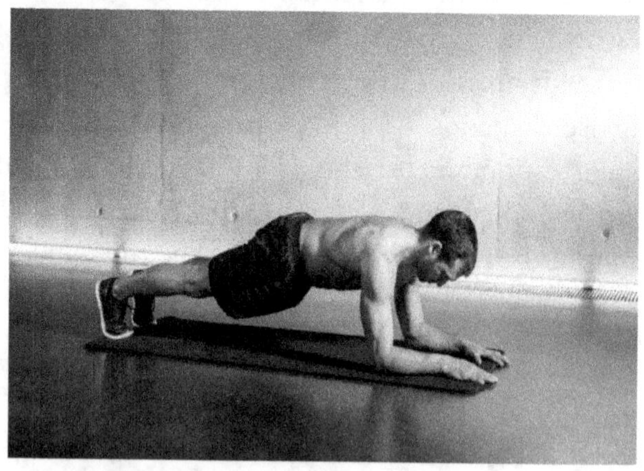

5. Jumping with knee up

This exercise is extremely powerful and fun and will help you to strengthen your entire body, including your heart. It is also a wonderful way to improve your agility.

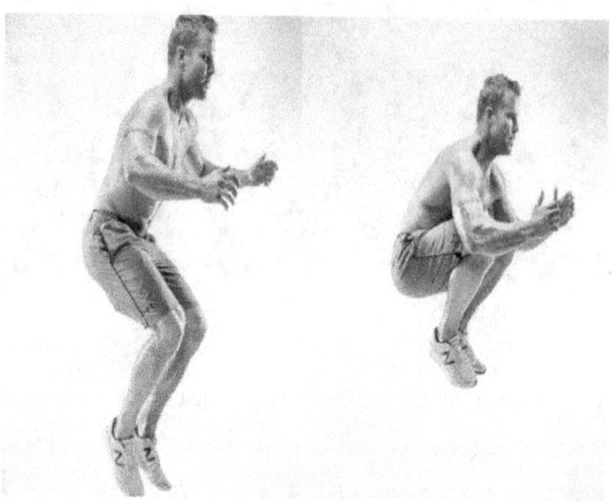

6. Weight lifting

When we repeatedly carry weight for a long period, our pelvic floor ends up exhausting and giving way overloaded.

Try to space out the times you need to carry weight and vary the load to give your muscles breaks.

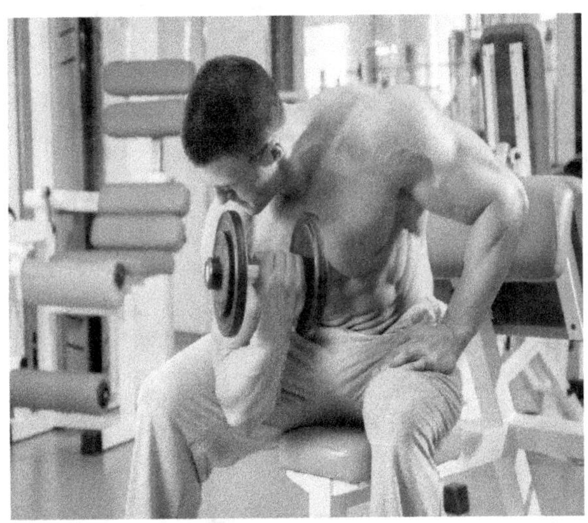

7. Declined bench press

The bench or board should incline to approximately 30 degrees. The exercise can be done on the fixed device, on the smith, or with free weights (which are more difficult).

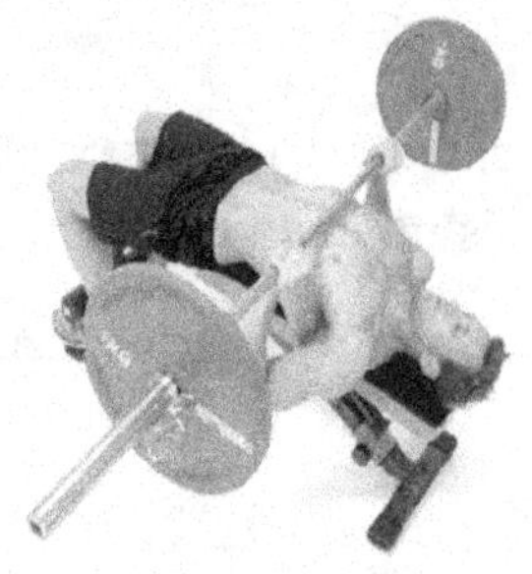

8. Declined flexion

Place your feet on a bench or any other support and flex your arms until your chest almost touches the floor. Perform the exercise with slow, focused movements.

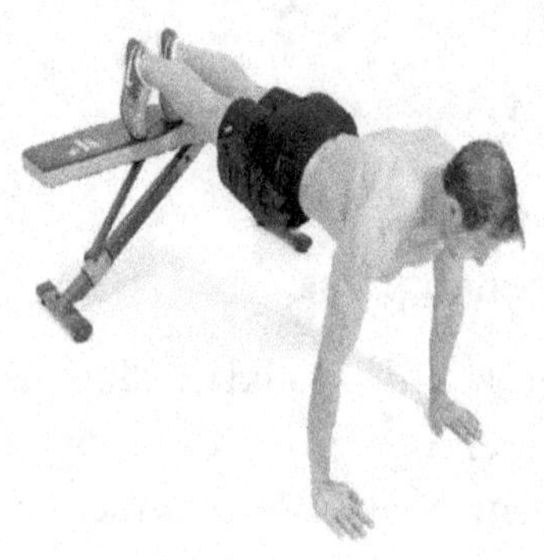

9. Hip lift

Support your feet on the floor with a bar on your lap and your back on a bench. Lift your hips until your body is straight from your shoulders to your knees and slowly lower yourself to the starting position. Pay attention to the alignment of the column. You can do it on the floor too, with a weight on your groin.

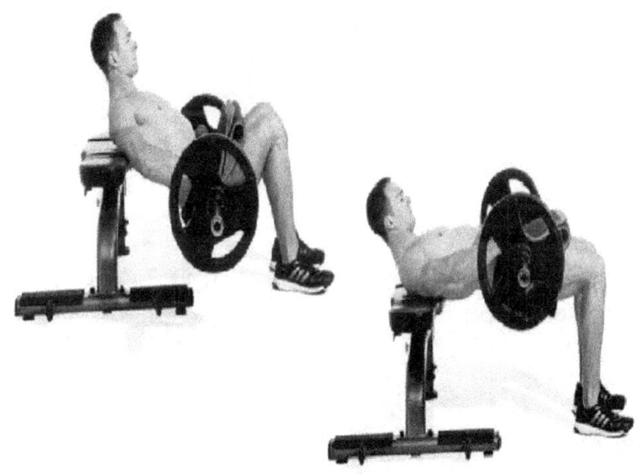

10. Sink and advance

With one foot in front and one in the back, lower your body until the back knee is close to the floor (both he and the front knee will be flexed at a 90-degree angle). Go back to the beginning. Your spine should always be straight. A variation of the sink is the advance, in which you "advance" by changing your legs during the strides. Increase the weights when exercise becomes easy.

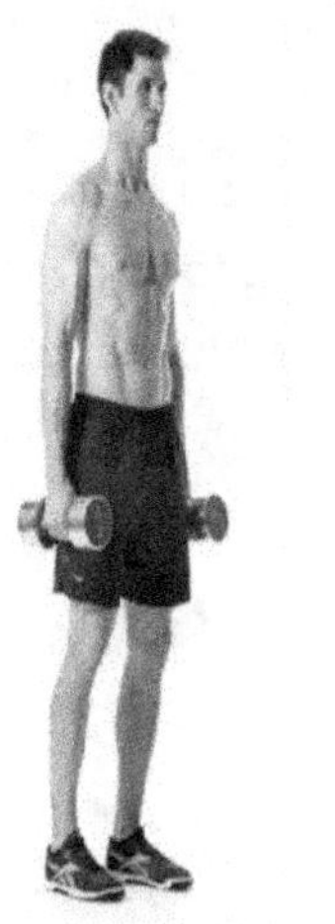

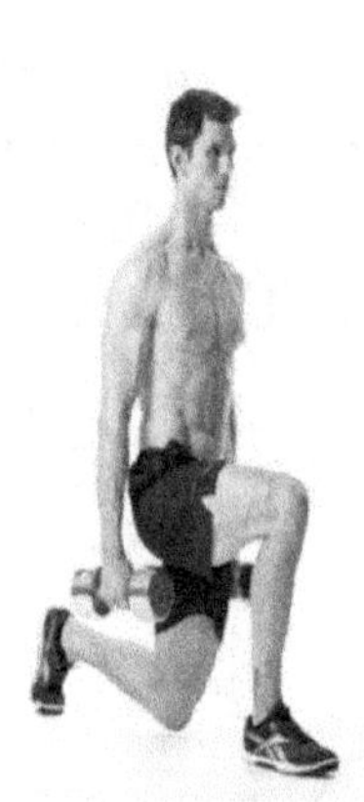

11. Lumbar extension

A small variation in position strongly activates the glutes. Just open your feet slightly outward, at a 45-degree angle to your heels. You will feel the difference.

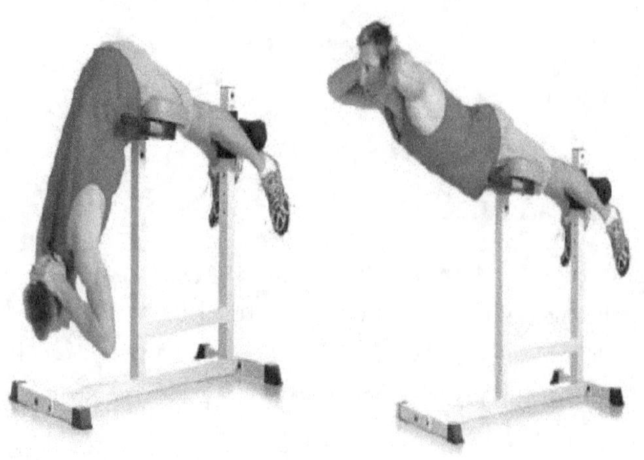

12. Kick in the handle

With your feet shoulder-width apart, attach one leg to the handle and bring it back, forcing the glutes to work. Keep your chest upright. Do the repetitions on one side and then switch.

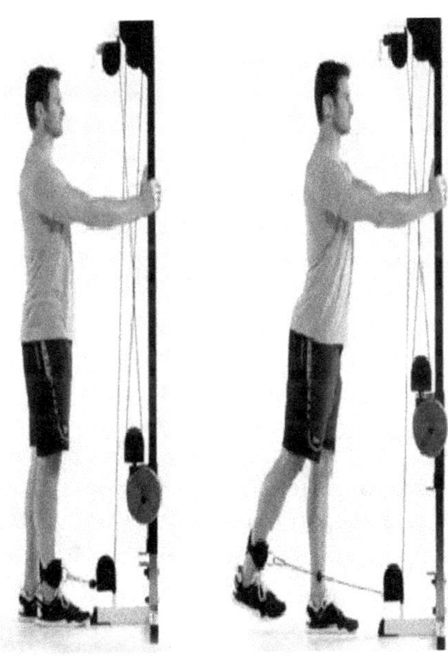

Muscle building supplements

Whether it's a classic, masculine, or bikini physique, it's tough to hit the stage after months of hard work and diet in the best shape of all time.

Your body has been through hell and your back, hunger, fatigue, and muscle aches are three things during your prep that make you immune to it too. Your supplement stack will help you overcome these obstacles and overcome workout plateaus. They not only help your body recover but also help build and maintain muscle during your bulk or cutting season.

Making sure you're consuming the best bodybuilding supplements can be the dividing line between first and second. If you put the work in, then your body deserves a helping hand too.

We've handpicked the best bodybuilding supplements the money can buy, backed by the science and why you need to add them to your stack if you're serious about competing.

Best supplements for bodybuilding

Wanting to get as big as possible or shredded to step out on stage? Get ready for muscle pumps and veins in places you never thought had veins. Take a look at the best supplements for bodybuilding below.

1. Whey Protein

Protein in general should become a stable part of your weight training regimen. Fuel your muscles with amino acids throughout the day or after training to help repair micro-tears caused by training.

Each type of protein you digest takes a different time to be broken down into amino acids to then stimulate protein synthesis. The faster you can stimulate this, the better.

For example, a chicken cutlet takes longer to break down and digest than a whey protein shake. Which is one of the reasons for consuming a post-workout shake. It is extremely important to ensure that your body receives protein instantly after a workout, as it helps jumpstart the recovery process as soon as possible.

If an athlete or bodybuilder consumes an insufficient amount of protein in their diet, they can develop a negative nitrogen balance, indicating protein catabolism, slow recovery (Phillips et al. 2011) and possibly, a waste of time. muscle wasting, injury, and even disease.

Of course, it depends on your height, weight, age, and gender. It can determine how much protein you need to eat. Recent research indicates that athletes may benefit from consuming approximately twice the RDA to maintain protein balance (Jager et al. 2017). The studies carried out by Witard et al. (2016), Jager et al. (2017), and Tipton et al. (2007), indicated that current evidence shows that, to optimize protein intake, it should be between 1.2 and 2.0 g per kg per day to stimulate protein synthesis and contribute to the muscle mass training.

However, as noted, different sources of protein are digested and absorbed at different rates, which can affect the protein you consume during the day, which can affect the body's catabolism and anabolism, and acute stimulation of muscle protein synthesis (Bucci et al. 2000). . So this should be taken into account when choosing what to do.

We've only scratched the surface of whey protein, which has benefits not only for bodybuilding but health and wellness as well.

2. Creatine Monohydrate

Creatine Monohydrate is hailed as the sacred supplement in bodybuilding. With the ability to boost energy, reduce fatigue, and aid in muscle and power gains, there's a reason all of your bodybuilding idols are using it daily.

Present in pre-workouts or consumed alone, creatine monohydrate is incredibly versatile and should be consumed if you are looking to build significant muscle mass.

Creatine is believed to be one of the most studied supplements on the market. For those studying creatine monohydrate and muscle gains, research has shown that creatine supplementation increases body mass during training (Williams, 1999), with typical increases of 1 to 2 kg for 4 to 12 weeks. training (Kreider, 2002).

The gains in muscle mass are said to be because creatine can allow our muscles to function at a higher intensity (Volek et al. 1999), thus allowing the athlete to train harder, which in turn results in more large adaptations to training and muscle hypertrophy (Olsen et al. 2006).

Creatine Monohydrate has shown very positive results for bodybuilders and is a natural supplement that you should add to your stack to reach your full potential. Creatine monohydrate helps increase phosphocreatine stores, which can then be used to produce more ATP, which is an essential energy source for strength training and high-intensity exercise.

3. BCAA

Branched Chain Amino Acid or BCAAs, as it is often called, is a popular supplement around the world. Used by the most elite athletes in your average clientele for their ability to build muscle. BCAAs are a mixture of amino acids made up of leucine, isoleucine, and valine. These amino acids all play an important role in our body and are more commonly referred to as the building blocks of muscles.

Amino acids are found in protein, however, BCAAs are simply a concentrated mixture of what you find there. You may have already heard of leucine and its main ability to stimulate protein synthesis. It does this by activating and stimulating our mTOR pathways. This is a regulator in our body which is linked to the health and growth of cells. When leucine stimulates the mTOR pathway, it sends signals to promote protein synthesis and muscle protein synthesis, which allow the body to repair and build muscle mass, helping you to recover and achieve significant gains.

BCAAs are used for 3 main principles in bodybuilding.

1) muscle growth.

2) Muscle pain.

3) Performance.

As a collective, these 3 will help you bring your best physique to the stage.

For example, one study found that protein synthesis was 22% higher in those who consumed a BCAA drink after training than in those who took a placebo (Whitard et al. 2014). BCAAs have also been observed to have positive reflections on muscle soreness. People who took BCAAs after leg workouts reported less muscle pain the next day after the placebo group. (Shimomura et al. 2010)

Taking a BCAA supplement at the right time is vitally important to getting the most out of it.

4. Caffeine

Caffeine has had a positive impact on increasing energy expenditure (number of calories burned) and may promote weight loss (Goldstein et al. 2010), which, if you need it for your competition, can help you lose weight. help: the edge by dropping the pounds.

In addition to improving your BMI, caffeine has had a positive impact on your performance. Although the following studies were done under a sports scenario, the principles are the same, as they can help you perform exercises at a higher intensity. The caffeine supplement drink has been found to improve speed, peak power, and average power in trained cyclists (Wiles et al. 2006). This was also observed in a similar study conducted by (Ivy et al. 2009) a time trial that showed performance improvements and repeated sprint performance in a separate study (Graham, 2001).

Caffeinated pre-workouts will give you the energy and motivation to start your workout, even if you don't quite feel up to it. With some cool new additions to the mix to help you with your workout, you won't be able to train without it the next time you go.

In addition to containing caffeine, an important ingredient, premium pre-workout powders also contain many energy and muscle-building ingredients that work synergistically and can often save you time instead of consuming a mixture of different. supplements. For example, the best pre-workouts will include BCAAs, beta-alanine, citrulline malate, creatine monohydrate, and glutamine. We will talk about some of their benefits below.

5. Beta-Alanine

For some, beta-alanine might be a supplement you haven't heard of, but chances are you've consumed it at some point if you've ever had a pre-workout blend. Beta-alanine is a non-essential amino acid and plays a role in the synthesis of carnosine. Carnosine is said to be one of the most important buffering substances in muscles, helping to reduce the chances of fatigue due to a build-up of lactic acid, which allows you to perform more and build muscle bigger. Simple science.

Studies have shown that by increasing carnosine levels while taking beta-alanine over 28 days (Harris et al 2009), this increase in carnosine in the body has shown an increase in the number of repetitions of the beta-alanine (Hoffman et al. 2009), increase lean body mass (Smith et al. 2009) and increase training performance (Hoffman et al. 2009). All of this put together shows the importance of beta-alanine supplementation when looking at bodybuilding or show preparation.

Having the ability to perform more reps at a high intensity will allow you to increase your overall performance. More reps can equate to a better contribution to increasing strength, and overall this causes more tears in the muscle fibers, which when repaired will result in bigger muscles.

Beta-alanine is often combined with other supplements to increase the chances of increasing muscle mass.

6. Citrulline Malate

Citrulline malate is a non-essential amino acid, and as described, it can be found in many high-end pre-workout supplements, but it can also be taken on its own. Citrulline malate is only found in very limited amounts in the body, but it is commonly known to be found in watermelon. We do not recommend that you eat a whole one before training, it is much easier to buy the supplement on its own.

Citrulline malate plays a vital role in the body. It is easily digested and absorbed by our bloodstream, which is then sent directly to our kidneys. Here, the citrulline malate is then converted to arginine at a better rate than it would be if you had just consumed the arginine itself. The arginine is then converted to nitric oxide, a powerful neurotransmitter that helps our blood vessels, but we'll cover that in more detail below.

There are three major benefits of consuming citrulline malate if you want to gain muscle mass and improve your workouts.

Increase in NO production

The world of sports nutrition is inundated with nitric oxide supplements, but the one that stood out from the crowd has always been citrulline malate. Nitric oxide plays a role in regulating blood flow, oxygen supply, glucose uptake, muscle firepower, and muscle growth, among other psychological benefits. This means that citrulline malate can dilate your blood vessels, allowing nutrients and other supplements to reach the muscles faster and easier. Not to mention that it will also give you a bigger pump and has also been shown to increase the rise in growth hormones after exercise (Seureda et al. 2010)

Reduces lactic acid

Thus, citrulline malate also plays a role in the urea cycle. The urea cycle is a system in the liver that helps release enzymes and convert and remove all wastes from the body, including lactic acid and ammonia. The accumulation of both, even in the most elite athletes, can cause extreme fatigue and even dementia. By consuming citrulline malate, you are helping to eliminate this excess waste, which helps limit the risk of the dreaded muscle cramps. Less muscle fatigue and muscle cramps equal more reps and better gains.

Increases recovery of ATP and phosphocreatine

Studies on citrulline malate have also shown significant positive effects on increasing the rate of ATP production and phosphocreatine recovery in the body after training (bendahan et al. 2009). ATP is a major key to energy production in the cell. This allows your muscles to work harder for longer which gives you a better chance of making those really big gains.

If we combine all of the above, you will understand why citrulline malate has become a force to be reckoned with. Because of these benefits now demonstrated by bodybuilding and athletic performance, citrulline malate has become THE ideal supplement for research to determine what more it can provide.

In one study, it was found that weightlifters who consumed at least 8g of citrulline malate before a workout could perform 54.92% more reps compared to those who consumed a placebo drink. Being able to perform more reps leads to the tearing of more muscle fibers, increased strength, and an overall increase in muscle size (Pérez-Guisado, 2010)

7. Glutamine

Glutamine is another amino acid (it seems to be the muscle that is currently growing). Again, these are often found in other supplements such as pre-workouts, but can also be consumed on their own. Glutamine plays a key role in protein metabolism, cell volumizer, and anabolism. This is especially important during the competitive cutting phase, as it helps to maximize your body's ability to maintain muscle when you start to lose body fat.

Although glutamine has many more benefits for the bodybuilding community than just maintaining muscle. Glutamine has also been shown to be extremely important for the immune system. When you exercise, your body is under a lot of stress and its immune system weakens, allowing bacteria and infections to take control. This would result in you getting sick and taking time out at the gym. The worst phrase you can say to any bodybuilder.

Studies have shown that if your body naturally produces less glutamine than it needs, then it could start breaking down protein stores, such as muscle, to release more of this amino acid (De-Souza et al., 1998), which would result in muscle wasting, weakness, and even illness if the lack of glutamine in the body becomes a regular occurrence. Similar studies have also found that a lack of glutamine in the body can compromise the immune system (Calder et al., 1999).

While glutamine is much easier to consume with supplements, you can also increase your intake through the foods you eat.

Muscle gain for female

Those who think that a gym is a place for men only are wrong. Women also want (and can!) To have a defined body and gain muscle mass. First of all, it is necessary to understand that women's training will be different from men's, precisely because of the biology of the woman's body. Thus, the diet to gain muscle mass also needs to be different.

The difference is good, as it fits your shape.

How to gain muscle growth

What do you think of perfect bodies? This is a topic that generates controversial opinions. But, when we talk about female hypertrophy, some misconceptions make her look at it negatively. It must be clarified that the term "increase in muscle mass" is not always related to muscles that are too large. This is because it also refers to the burning of fats and the definition of the body.

This practice aims to increase muscle and contributes to the preservation of the functioning of metabolism in general. The ideal fat percentage for women seeking female hypertrophy is between 20% and 24%.

To arrive at this body composition takes dedication and patience. So, whatever your goal of hypertrophy, get to know the 7 tips we have separated in this post and put them into practice.

1. Train your whole body and vary the exercises

When only part of the body is trained, there is a significant reduction in the quality of bodybuilding. That is, training the whole body optimizes the results. Also, at certain times, you need to exercise with higher loads and fewer repetitions.

6 to 12 repetitions with more challenging weights are recommended. The fact is that the muscles need to be

stressed frequently for the muscle fiber regeneration process to take place.

Training in this way, there will be an increase in lean mass, decrease in fat, and, consequently, greater muscle definition. Conversely, when the stimuli are always the same, the body remains undeveloped and there is no hypertrophy.

2. Always include protein in meals

Your diet needs to be aligned with your goal. Protein acts on muscle building. Therefore, when you are training regularly, you need to ensure that you are ingesting it in an amount sufficient for tissue recovery and definition.

Protein consumption varies depending on your goal and lifestyle. For hypertrophy, it is recommended to consume two grams of protein daily per kilogram of body weight. However, as important as the quantity, is the distribution of the substance throughout the day: divide the two grams between your main meals.

3. Use supplementation

Often, protein consumption through food is not enough. In these cases, it is important to supplement with Whey Protein, usually taken after training or as a way to fill the nutritional deficit of meals low in the protein of the day.

But one must be aware that supplementation does not work miracles. The ideal is to include the product within a diet plan so that you have more results when it comes to gaining muscle mass.

Another advantage of supplements is practicality. With the exhaustive routine that we have today, making use of supplementation is a way of maintaining the diet and consuming the amount of protein prescribed, as it is easy to transport and consume Whey Protein.

In addition to Whey Protein, creatine also deserves special mention. It is of great value for increasing muscle volume when it is inserted into a diet and the instructions for use are respected. Looking for a sports nutritionist ensures that your goal is achieved faster.

4. Get adequate rest

Sleep and rest mustn't be neglected. When the person is tired, in addition to not being able to exercise properly, he still has unregulated hormones. Besides, muscles need a certain period of rest to recover and develop.

During sleep, our body releases hormones that help in gaining muscle mass. It can be said that it is the moment that the body uses to recover from the stress caused by the overload of the exercise series. But, for this to happen, it is recommended to sleep 6 to 8 hours daily.

Satisfactory sleep enhances the burning of fats, enhances muscle definition, regulates metabolism, and balances the body, making female hypertrophy faster.

5. Consume appropriate carbohydrates and lipids

In addition to the proteins already mentioned, a good diet should contain the proper amount of carbohydrates and lipids. Many women think that they need to stop consuming them, which is a big mistake. Without them, there will be serious problems in muscle development.

Lipids collaborate for hormonal production, thermal regulation, and positive nitrogen balance in tissues. In turn, carbohydrates provide energy. So, don't miss your diet of eggs, avocado, seeds, olive oil, sweet potatoes, brown bread, brown or white rice, yams, beans, quinoa, and oats.

6. Eat a lot

One of the most common mistakes that women make and that makes it difficult to gain muscle mass and, consequently, female hypertrophy is to eat little. Building muscle requires energy.

To increase lean mass, you need to consume more calories than you expend. However, it is necessary to eat good foods, such as those mentioned above. Consuming too little food will cause the metabolism to slow down, making weight loss and maintenance difficult. The excess calories, in addition to the workouts, favor the increase of muscles.

Another important tip about food is not to skip meals. Strictly follow the meal plan and eat 5 to 6 meals a day ensures that the necessary amounts of calories are consumed.

7. Hydrate yourself

When we talk about female hypertrophy, we immediately remember flat stomachs. However, one of the biggest complaints of women is the swelling caused by fluid retention. Most of the time, this swelling appears in the abdomen.

Drinking plenty of water helps to eliminate impurities and does not retain liquid. But it is not only that because, in the composition of our muscles, but it is also always present. Therefore, for muscle cells to grow and muscle mass to gain, water is needed.

Also, water is responsible for homeostasis, which consists of the processes of breathing, digestion, and excretion, essential for maintaining the body's balance. 35 ml of water per kg of weight is recommended for healthy adults.

Anyway, female hypertrophy aims at weight loss with muscle definition. To achieve a shapely body, it is necessary to train all muscle groups, follow a balanced diet and not neglect rest and hydration. These practices, taken together, will give you the body you want.

Exercises to build muscle

Before starting to perform the training, it is important to warm up to decrease the risk of injury and speed up the metabolism, in addition to stimulating conditioning and resistance to complete the training. So, to warm up, you can jump rope, run on the spot or do jumping jacks, for example, for about 30 seconds to 1 minute.

Besides, it must be kept in mind that the exercises in this plan must be performed 2 times for about 30 seconds and the rest must be 15 seconds. Between each group of exercises, the rest time should also be 15 seconds to allow muscle recovery.

1- Romanian Deadlift with Kettlebell

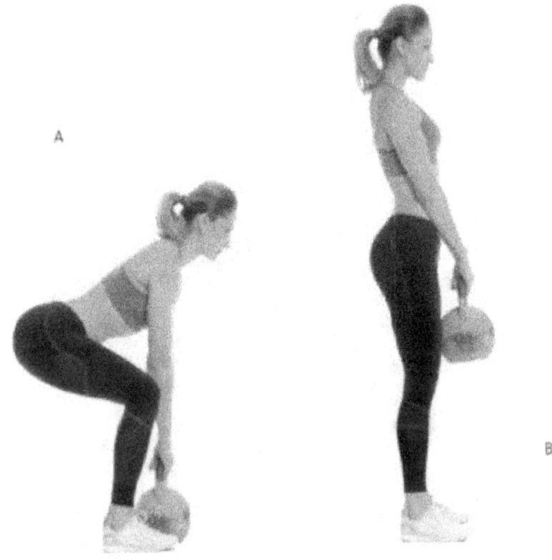

The deadlift is a powerful exercise that works the entire back of your body, but especially your glutes and hamstrings.

Perform the exercise with your feet aligned with your hips, and your leg slightly bent.

Hold the kettlebell between your feet, and lower and lift your torso with the kettlebell in your hands. Do five sets of eight reps.

2- L-Sit

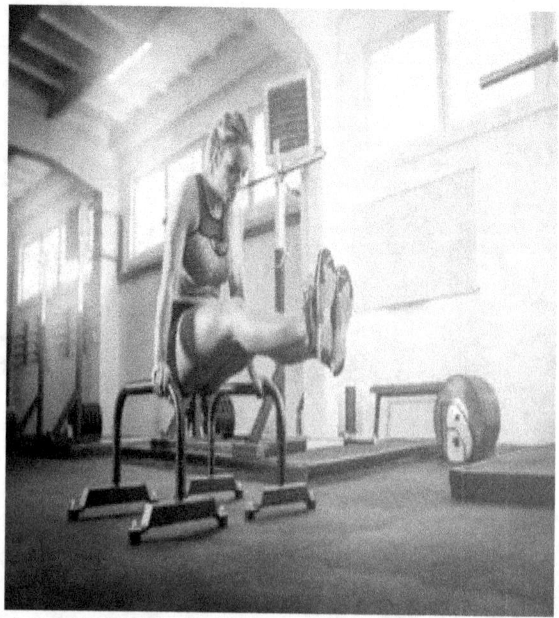

This challenging exercise can be modified for beginners, but no matter which version you do, you will feel your core screaming until the end.

Place push-up bars on both sides of your body, around the width of your shoulders.

With one hand on each bar, step off the floor and lift your legs to your hip, keeping your legs straight.

For beginners, you can bend your knees to facilitate this movement. Do four sets of 20 seconds.

3- Curved Row

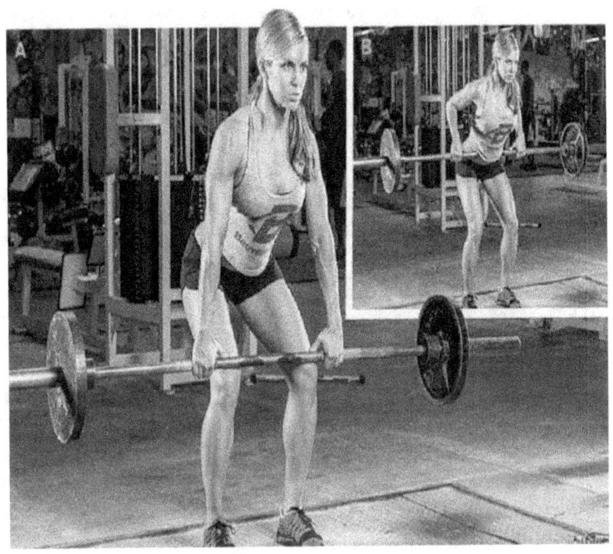

Many women leave iron-pulling exercises out of their routine. But it is important to add these types of exercises to your workouts to achieve a balanced body.

Position your feet in line with your hips and knees, slightly bent.

Make a grip on the bar with spacing equal to the width of the shoulders.

With the back of your hands facing up, tilt your torso forward at a 45-degree angle to the floor, then pull the bar up until it touches your chest.

Keep your spine straight, and lower the bar with your arms extended to the floor. Do four sets of eight reps.

4- Kettlebell Swings

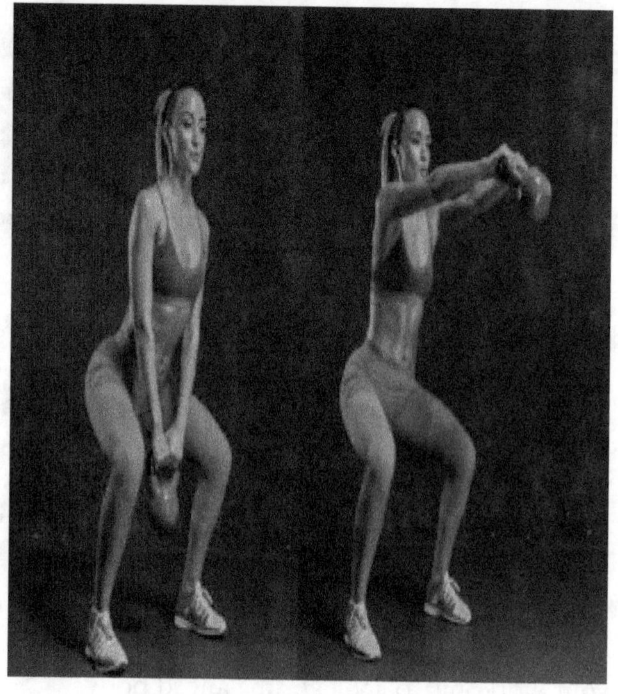

This kettlebell exercise is a full-body movement that looks easy to perform, but it isn't.

So, start with a lighter weight to feel how far your body can go before choosing a heavier and more challenging weight.

Standing upright, hold the kettlebell with both hands.

With the kettlebell falling between your legs, push your hips forward, bringing the kettlebell up to eye level.

Keep your arms straight with a slight bend at the elbows. Perform four sets of 12 reps.

5- Flexion

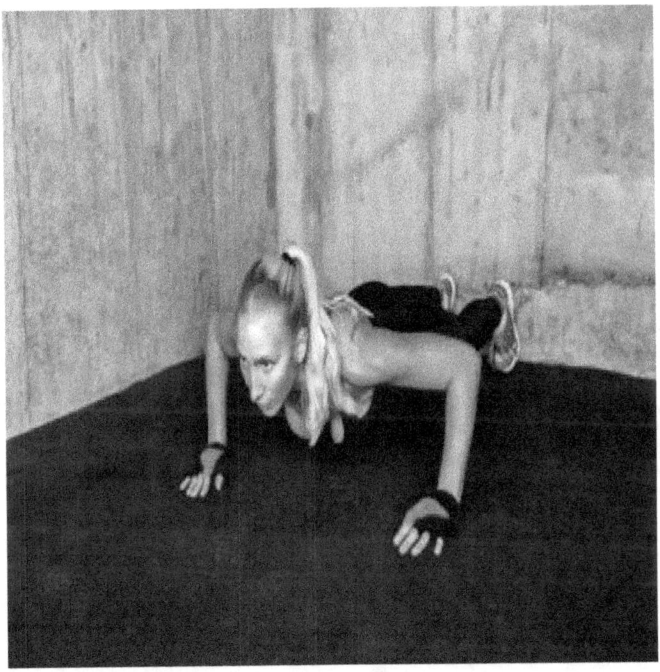

Last but not least, flexion!

One of the most common exercises and also one of the most effective in strengthening the entire body.

On a mat, lie on your stomach. With your body stretched, support your hands on the floor in line with your shoulders, raising and lowering your body with the strength of your arms.

Do four sets of eight reps.

You can still get a better result if you do all these exercises together, on the same circuit. But always count on the help of your coach.

Ready to face this challenge, and get your body in shape?

30 days diet plan

The diet to increase muscle mass includes strategies such as consuming more calories than you expend, increasing the amount of protein during the day, and consuming good fats. In addition to the reinforced diet, it is also important to do regular workouts that require a lot of muscle mass, as the hypertrophy stimulus is passed on to the body.

It is also important to remember that to gain lean and lose fat at the same time, one should avoid the consumption of sugar, white flour, and processed products, as they are the main stimulators of fat production in the body.

Here are some sample diet choices that you can use to create your own personalized 30 days meal plan for muscle growth.

Snack:	Day 1	Day 2	Day 3
Breakfast	2 slices of brown bread with egg and cheese + 1 cup of coffee with milk	1 chicken and cheese tapioca + 1 glass of cocoa milk	1 glass of sugar-free juice + 1 omelet with 2 eggs and chicken
Morning snack	1 fruit + 10 chestnuts	1 natural yogurt with	1 mashed banana with

	or peanuts	honey and chia seed	oats and 1 tablespoon peanut butter
Lunch dinner	4 tablespoons of rice + 3 tablespoons of beans + 150 g of grilled duckling + raw salad of cabbage, carrots, and peppers	1 piece of salmon + boiled sweet potatoes + sautéed salad with olive oil	Ground beef pasta with wholegrain pasta and tomato sauce + 1 glass of juice
Afternoon snack	1 yogurt + 1 whole chicken sandwich with curd	fruit smoothie with 1 tablespoon of peanut butter + 2 tablespoons of oats	1 cup of coffee with milk + 1 crepe filled with 1/3 can of tuna

By following all the rules and exercises, you can achieve the desired result in 30 days.

Good luck!

Chapter Five

Home & Gym Workout

Physical exercise is essential to maintain health and also the opportunity to define the body and lose some measures. The important thing is to keep moving.

It is important, before beginning the exercises, to consult a doctor to check if you can perform physical activities.

And is it worth training at home? If your goal is to have more convenience and savings, you are on the right track. It is an opportunity to save on gym fees.

How to train at home

Training at home is practical, but it takes some attitudes for the training to have results. First, it is necessary to leave laziness aside, as it is useless to buy fitness equipment and after a while, leave everything aside. You need to be excited to continue training. Have a goal, so it's easier to stay motivated. And speaking of that:

What is your goal?

Keep in mind if you want to lose weight, strengthen your muscles or 2, as each device has a different function. This makes it easier to choose fitness equipment to train at home.

Set a budget

Decide how much you want to spend so you don't get out of budget and make the right choice of gym equipment to train at home.

Reserve a space to perform the exercises

There is no need for a large space, it should just be enough for you to move around during your workout.

Do not do the activities or use the devices on your own without knowledge

A professional specialized in-home training knows exactly how to use the equipment correctly, thus avoiding future injuries.

Time and patience

It is essential to emphasize that the objective is not achieved quickly, it is necessary to have the patience to wait for the results.

Stretching is important

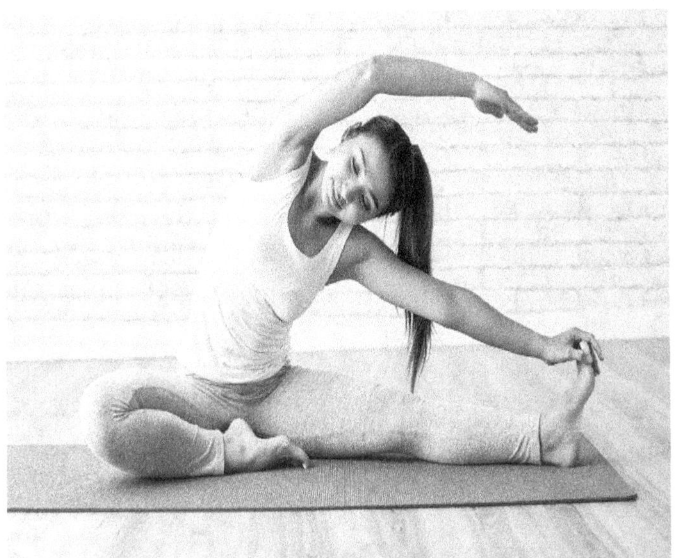

Before facing any training, the body needs to be prepared to receive the exercise. Stretching should be done before and in some cases afterward (post-workout) to allow relaxation, being done lightly without harming the muscle worked. In this case, the opinion of a specialist is also interesting.

Training intensity

Each activity has a level, if it has been rusty for a long time, start slowly and evolve as your body gets used to it.

Proper clothing

Opt for flexible models that make it easy to do activities.

Food is a great ally

Before exercise, eat light foods to avoid disrupting your performance. Never exercise without eating. And the opposite also serves, nothing to eat too much, can cause indigestion.

It is important to know that exercise alone does not work miracles, so it is important to have a correct diet to get the expected result. Consult an expert to find the ideal diet for you.

Hydrate yourself during workouts

Always keep a small bottle of water on hand, as you train your body to sweat.

Correct breathing

When it comes to running, the right breathing is essential for the proper progress of the exercise. Breathe through your nose and abdominal, for example, inhale at the time to go up and exhale on the way down.

Set the time to work out

The morning period is more suitable, as it speeds up the metabolism and gives more disposition during the day, but it is important to respect the defined time regardless of the period (morning, afternoon, or night).

Sound to motivate

Prefer the dance playlists to give a gas during the training.

TV and mobile

Avoid these devices while you are training, as they are two items that can be distracting and so you end up not performing the activity correctly.

Call someone to train

It is a way to stay motivated in your goal because at home several temptations can deviate from the exercises.

Fitness equipment for training at home

See the fitness devices to train at home and stay in shape!

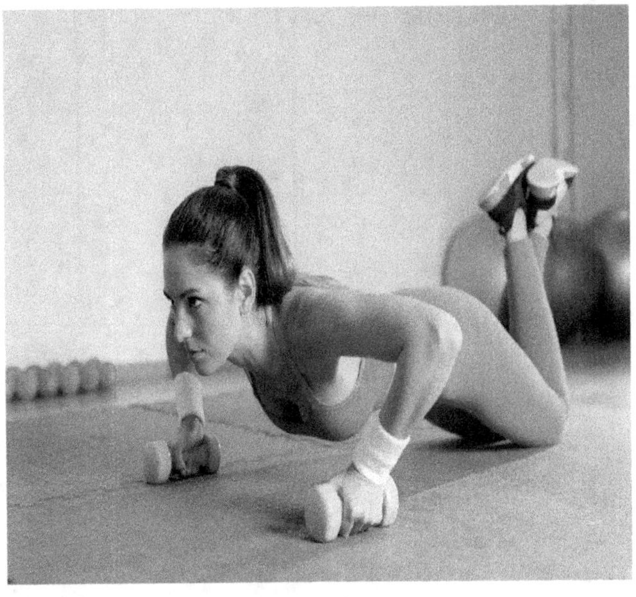

Having a gym at home has the advantage of not having to wake up too early or worry about commuting, but it will require discipline to continue training.

For those who do not have the habit of training, the idea is to opt for functional and basic equipment. As you evolve you can buy more complex equipment, so you don't run the risk of giving up quickly. Therefore, in the beginning, it is important to start slowly to get used to the body.

Now if you already have the experience, it's nice to choose multifunctional equipment that is versatile or allows different activities in a single product.

Aerobic machines are indicated for those who want to lose weight and to reduce fats that assist in cardiac, respiratory, and elastic activity. Find out below the fitness devices to train at home and make the best choice.

Exercise Bike

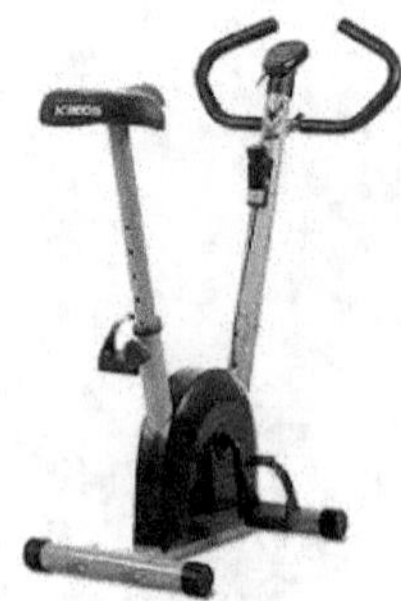

It is the activity that works the cardiac part, perfect for aerobic training.

Elliptic

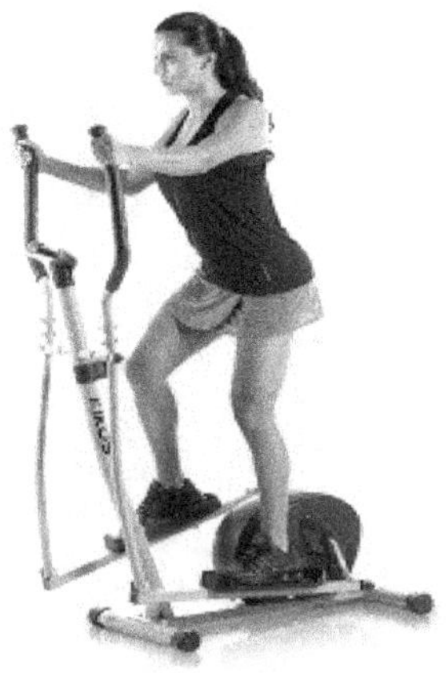

It is used in both aerobic and body-defining activities.

Bodybuilding Station

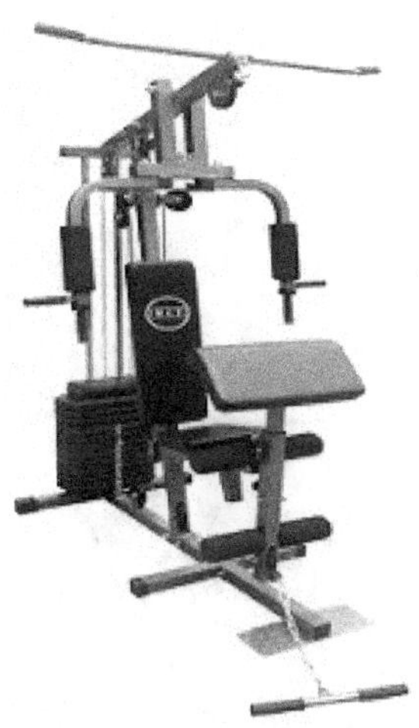

It is the most expensive device on the list, but before choosing, check your goal. Because it has different models, from the simplest to the complete equipment for all parts of the body. If you have space and can invest in multiple stations, buy without fear.

Running machine

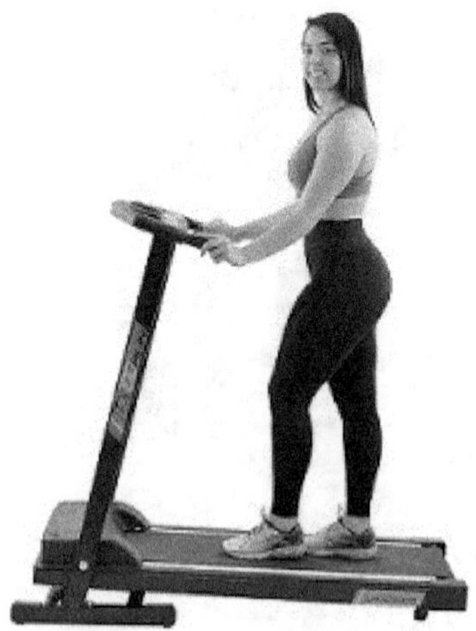

One of the most used devices in the gym. If you have space at home, it is worth the investment in the treadmill.

Walk simulator

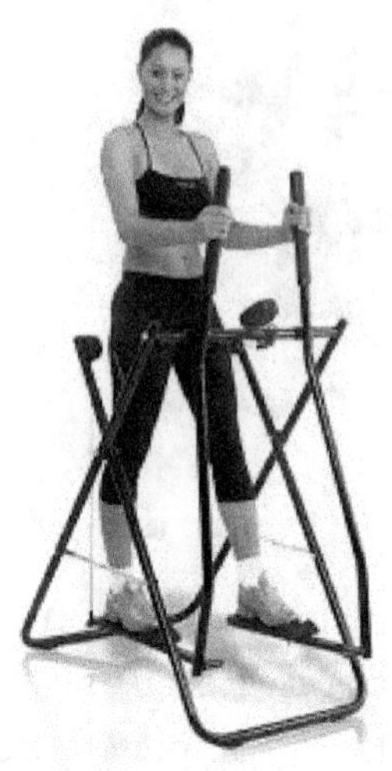

According to the name the goal is to walk, but it doesn't have as much impact as walking on the treadmill, for example. It is also worth it for its low cost. It has more compact models that make it easier to store, being one of the options of fitness devices to train at home.

Abdominal Tract

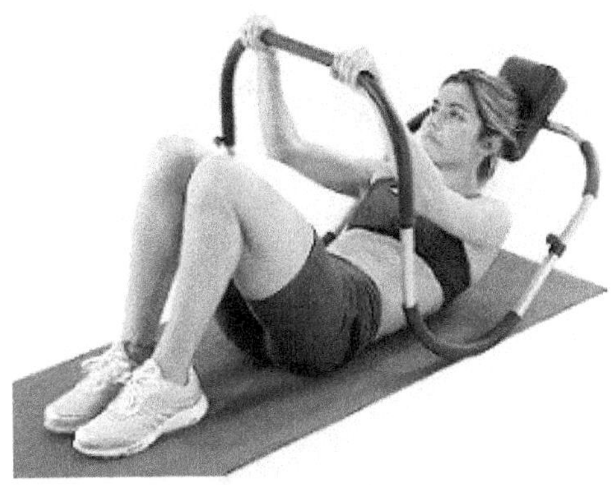

Helps reduce fat in the belly area.

Abdominal Wheel

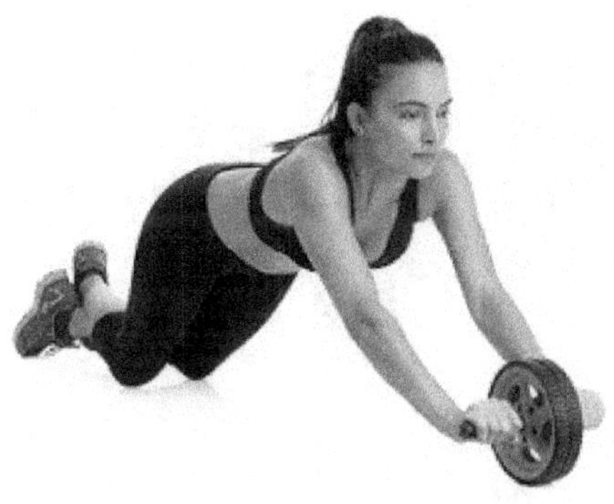

It has the same function as the abdominal apparatus, but it is a cheaper option.

Dumbbells / Ring

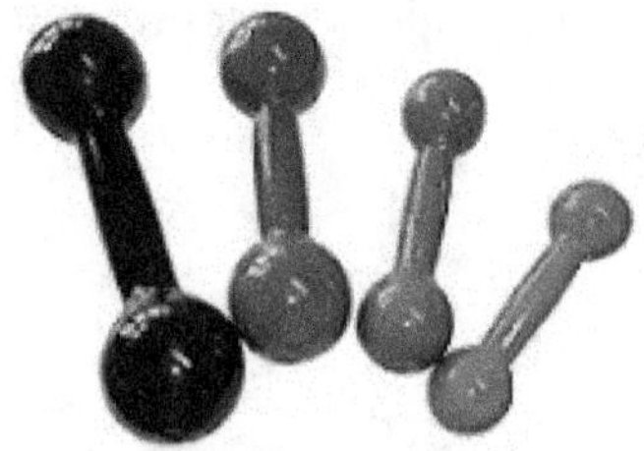

Weights for working arms, shoulders, and back.

Kettlebell

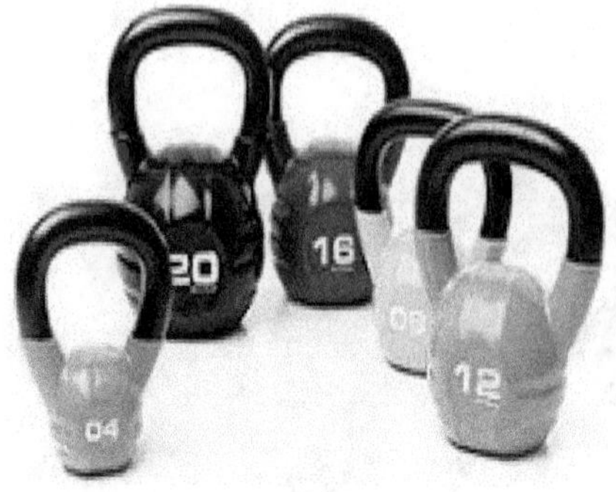

It has the same function as dumbbells, but the lower limbs work like glutes and legs.

Swiss Ball / Fitball / Gym Ball

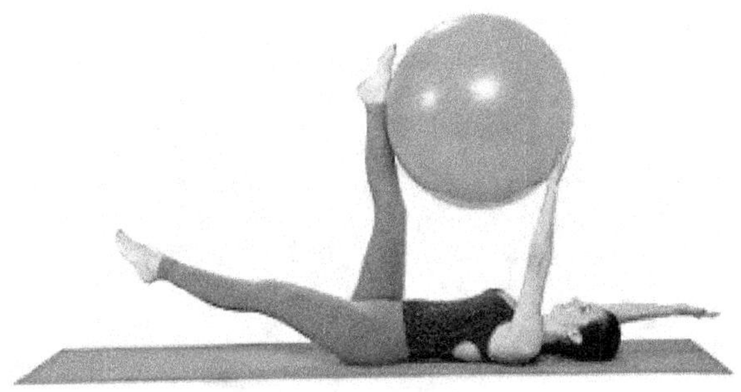

Another versatile item for training and can accompany a pump to fill.

Medicine Ball

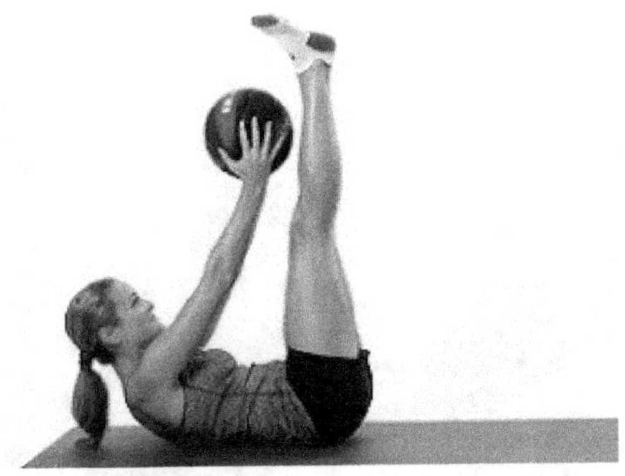

Unlike the Swiss ball, the medicine ball is a weighted ball that helps to work the muscles.

Jump / Trampoline

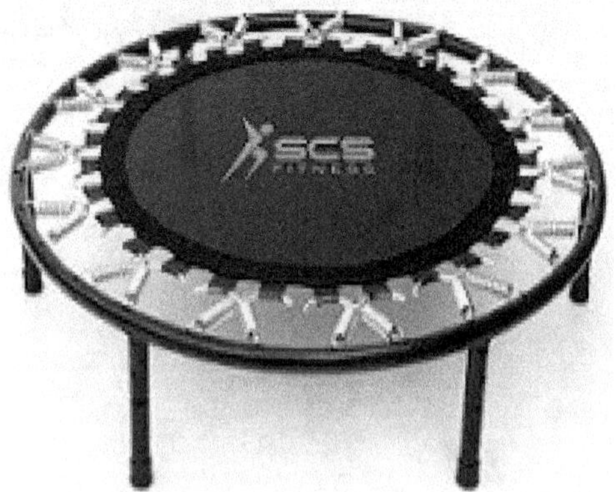

The trampoline is another option for fitness equipment to train at home. It is perfect for aerobic activities that use music to make your use more exciting.

Shin guards

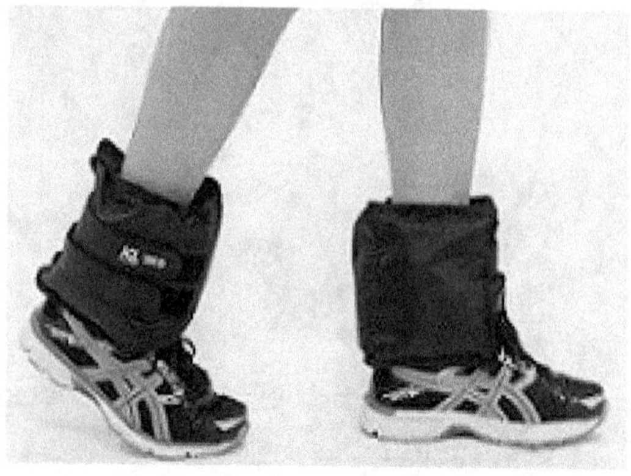

Start activities with 2kg shin guards for each leg.

Elastic Extender / Suspension Tape

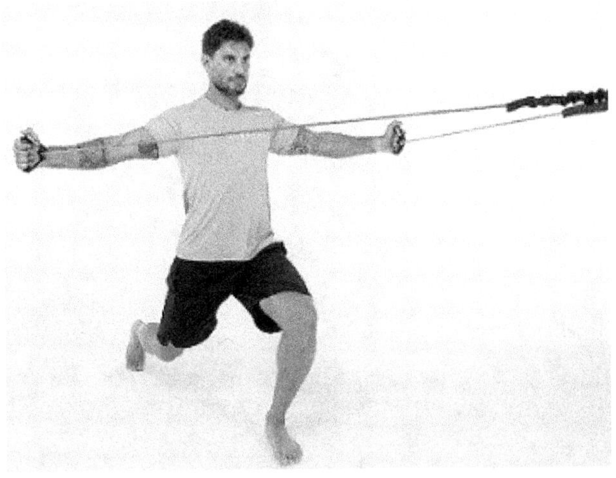

It serves activities that require difficulty, but that allow strengthening.

Mini Band / Elastic Band

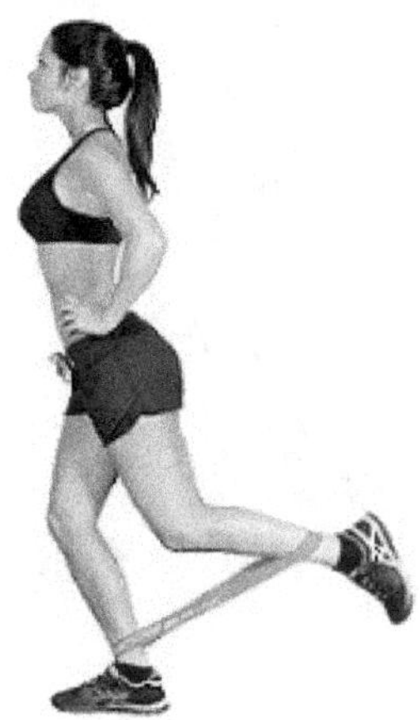

It is indicated for exercises on lower limbs, squats, and push-ups.

Ladder of Agility

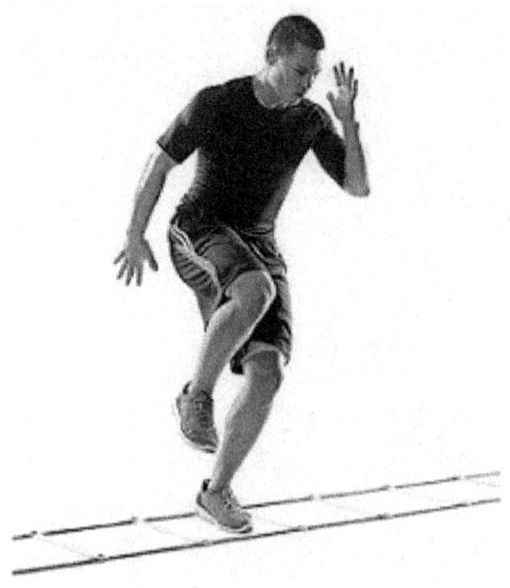

It allows the elaboration of several exercises for burning fat and slimming, but it needs space for execution.

Step

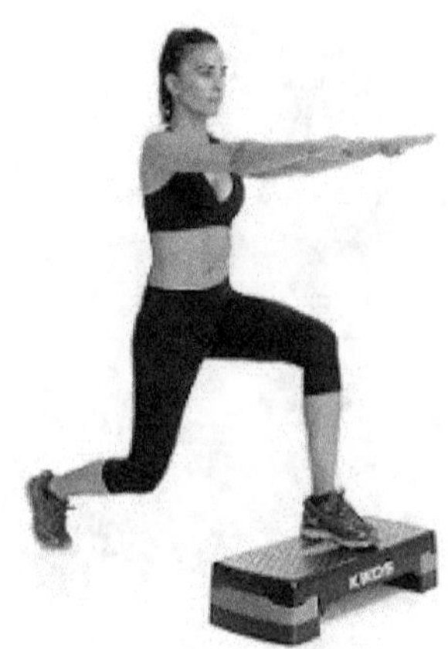

If you enjoy aerobic activities, the step is essential and low cost. Increase the sound and good training.

Slide Board / Sliding Platform

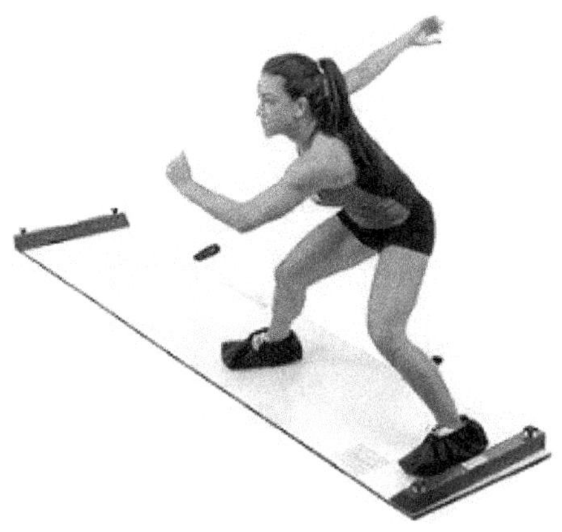

Another item that serves to tone the entire body, in addition to allowing activities such as pilates, for example.

Door Bar

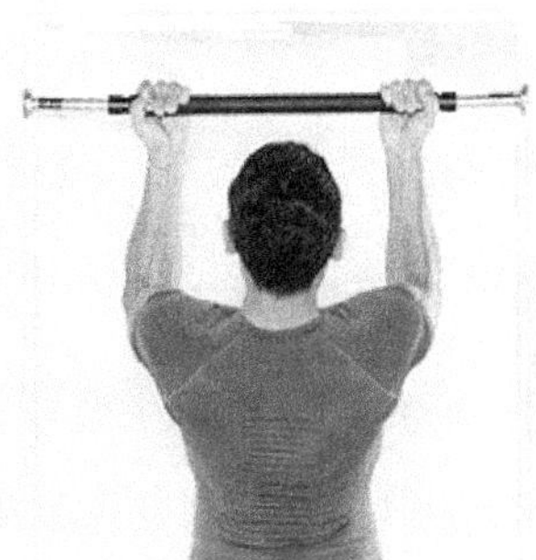

Uses body weight to strengthen.

Rope

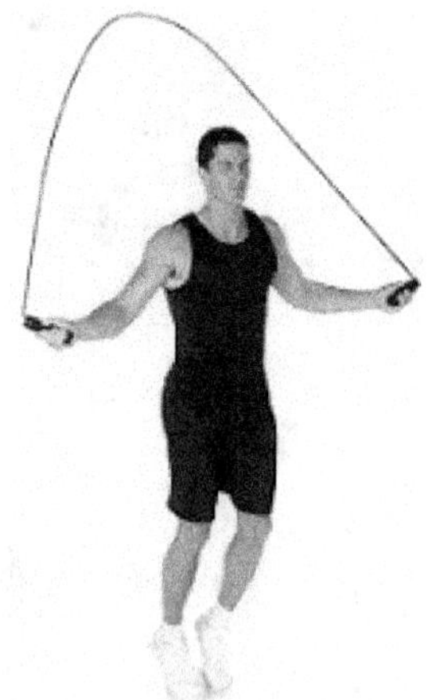

Skipping rope is aerobic training that works the whole body.

Flexion Support

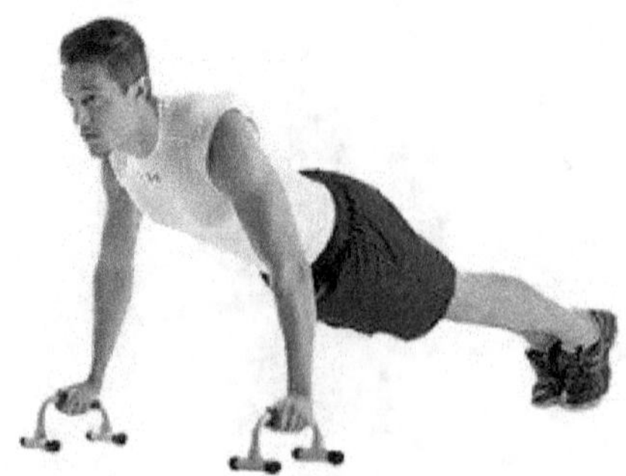

It helps when doing push-ups, with more intense movements that help define arms, back, and chest.

Mattress

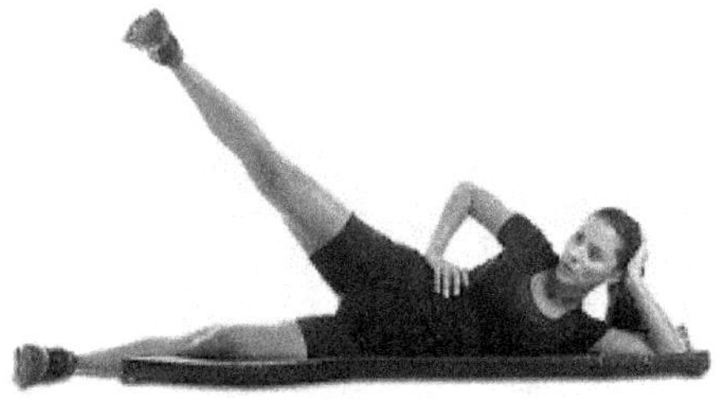

Essential item for training at home, as most exercises the mat is used, such as stretching.

Why do gym?

Increase in mood

Have you noticed that the more we stand still, the more we want to stand still? Despite being a natural tendency of the body, you can be willing to move around starting physical exercises.

At first, it may seem difficult to overcome laziness or tiredness after a long day of work or study to exercise. However, when you take the first step and overcome this initial difficulty, you will see that, with regularity, you will be more and more willing to leave home, gaining breadth and motivation to overcome your limits more and more.

If you have difficulty waking up early or feel discouraged during the day, you will certainly find that, after adapting to physical exercises, you will feel more willing to develop other daily activities, both at home and at work.

Higher quality of life

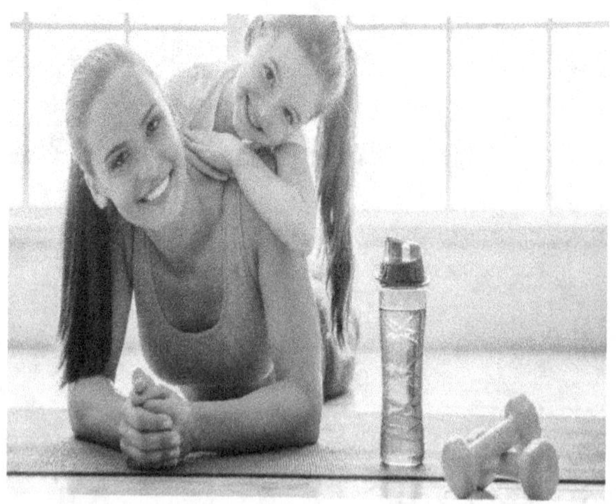

Going to the gym and developing the proposed physical exercises can make you happier! That's because, in general, moving regularly causes chemical reactions that generate an explosion of substances in the body, such as endorphin - one of the hormones linked to pleasure and satisfaction. These hormones affect fighting problems such as depression, in addition to providing greater well-being to practitioners.

All of this will provide a significant improvement in your quality of life, also increasing your agility, attention, and cognitive ability, as well as your interpersonal relationships.

Improvement in social life

Unlike training alone, at home, for example, gyms provide interaction with different people, which can directly influence your mental health and mood.

In gyms, in addition to teachers who, on several occasions, end up nurturing a closer relationship with students, you can meet people with similar goals to yours and find a training partner, creating a friendly and companionable environment.

Even if you are a more introverted person or you like to exercise focused on executing the movement, the simple act of giving a good day to different people or talking to a personal person provides a change in social life.

Health Gain

Physical exercise has several health benefits, in addition to being an important ally in the fight against obesity, which brings several complications. By regularly getting aroused, the body becomes more resistant and immune, avoiding infectious diseases (such as a cold or flu) and even acting to improve bronchitis or asthma.

In addition to the aesthetic issue, since attending the gym contributes to weight loss and lean mass gain, physical activities also:

- they work by improving physical conditioning ;
- increase cardiovascular capacity;
- fight problems related to diabetes;

- reduce cholesterol and hypertension, which reflects a lower risk of heart problems;
- increase body mobility;
- prevent osteoporosis;
- improve joints;
- fight depression, stress, and anxiety ;
- regulate the production of some hormones;
- stimulate healthy lifestyle habits, such as eating better and avoiding alcoholic beverages.
- That is, when you exercise you are investing in yourself, in your health, and your quality of life.
- **Increased confidence and self-esteem**

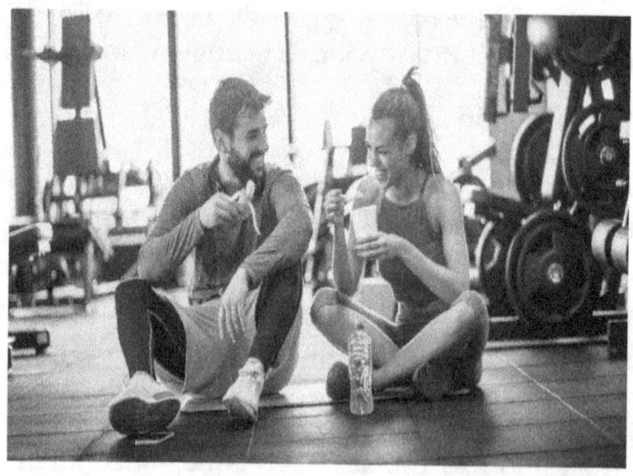

In addition to all the benefits listed so far, exercising at a gym contributes to the improvement of confidence and self-esteem, since, when we take physical activity seriously, we establish a goal and go in search of achieving it.

Upon reaching the goal, the feeling is of accomplishment, increasing confidence in our capacity. The improvement in self-esteem comes as a result of this process and of being at ease with yourself.

Things to consider before choosing a gym

Not every gym is the same, and not all are for you. See how to choose the right gym for your needs and enjoy your training even more!

Choosing the ideal gym is not choosing the most expensive, the biggest, the most beautiful, one of your friends or the first one you find - it may be a combination of some of these things, but it is also much more than that.

Before enrolling in any gym, you need to ask yourself a few questions - which include things like "Am I going to feel good here?"; "Can I pay for this gym?" among several others.

Academia is not "all the same"!

Choosing the right gym is essential to ensure that you reach your goals, have the desired results, enjoy training, have no injuries, among many other things.

Also, if you are going to take training seriously, your gym will be almost a second home - or at least a place where you will spend a considerable part of your routine.

That is why you need to think hard before enrolling. The right (or wrong) choice can define the future of your workouts. Want to see how to do this? Then read:

1- Have a clear objective

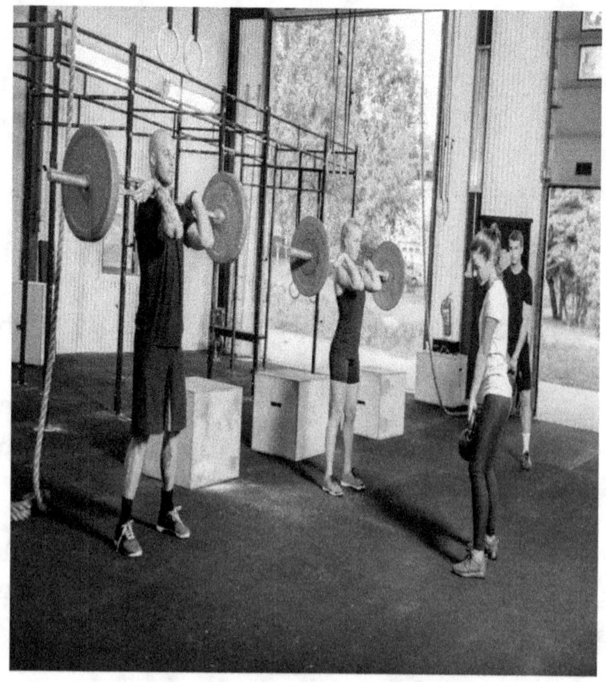

Its objective is a fundamental part of the choice process.

Do you want to be a professional athlete? A bodybuilder? Just want to look better and healthier? Want to enter obstacle and resistance races? Do CrossFit?

Each of these goals - and all thousands of others - has its own specific needs. Searching the gym with the right equipment, specialized teachers, among other characteristics that vary according to the modality, is a fundamental step.

Knowing where you want to go, and what you need to achieve your goal, will certainly eliminate some gyms from your list.

2- Location

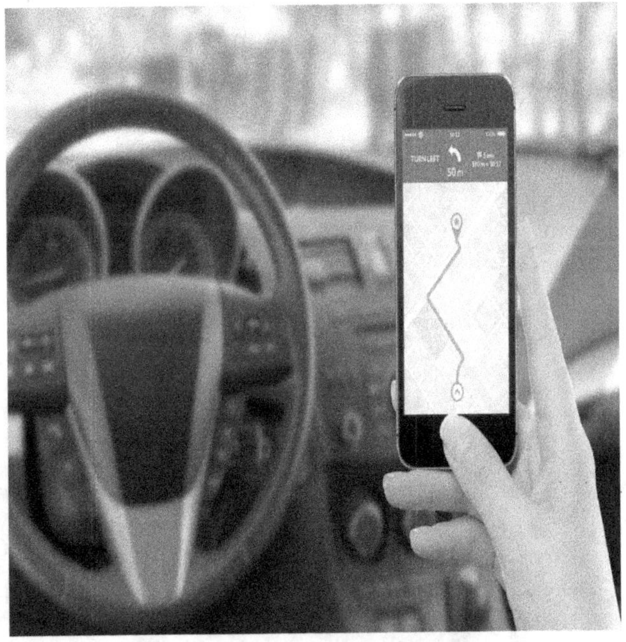

You can't train in a place where you take longer to arrive than you train. At the same time, the nearest gym is not always the one you get to the fastest.

Especially in large cities, you need to assess whether there is parking or parking spaces for cars - or, in the case of public transport, whether there are subways, trains or bus stops nearby.

Besides, it is also important to consider ease of access. Eventually, the gym closest to your home forces you to take a stroll through a region that lives with traffic.

Try to find an easily accessible gym. Otherwise, you are likely to miss a few days of training out of laziness or simply being unable to arrive on time.

3- Make "test-drives"

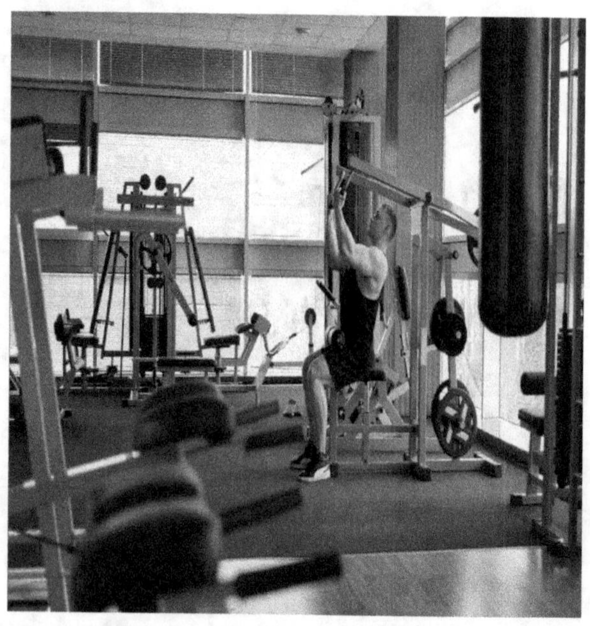

Almost every gym offers at least one free class for new students. Make use of this opportunity! Test before you buy!

This is important because, in general, gyms offer huge discounts for long plans - 6 or 12 months - and it isn't worth committing to paying that much gym time without making sure you're going to use it.

The test-drive is important not only for you to know the environment, the teachers, and the equipment, but also to test the arrival and departure times, the cleanliness and conservation of the place, among many other things.

When taking the test, remember to review all the details, and don't just go for a regular workout. It is the future of your training that will be at stake!

4- Check the equipment

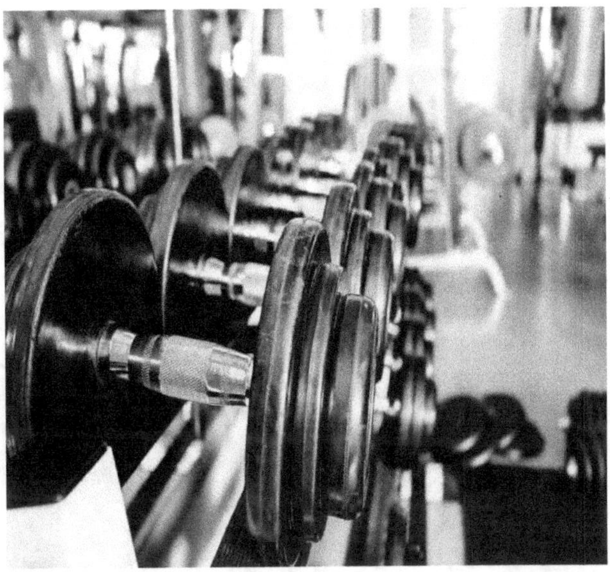

Having the most modern equipment is a positive point. But this is not the most important thing.

Especially because, it doesn't help the gym to have ultra-futuristic equipment, charge more for it, and you never even get close to them.

Check the number of dumbbells, bench presses, bars, power racks, and everything you are going to use. Nothing is more boring than going out to train and your session lasts three times as long because you had to wait to "wander" a piece of equipment in each series.

Another important point: the size of the site. Does the equipment stick together? Do people have to fight for space? All of this must be taken into account.

5- Energy and environment

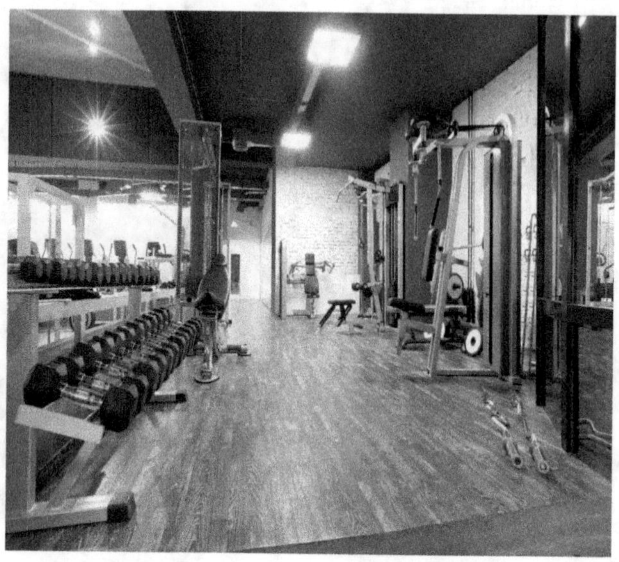

It may seem silly, but the energy of the place can directly affect your income.

A very noisy gym, for example, takes away concentration. An empty gym, very "cozy", can make you bored and even lazy.

Pay attention to things like the volume of ambient music, lighting, the number of people, the good (or bad) will of teachers and staff ... believe me: it does interfere with your routine.

It is also important to check hygiene and services: are the changing rooms good? Clean? Does the gym have drinking fountains working? Shower? All of this can influence your well-being.

6- Goers

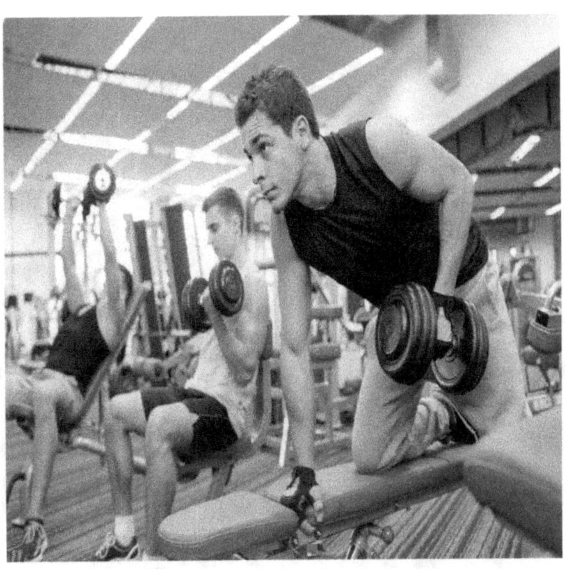

This is not so easy to detect on the first visit, but it is important. And it is valid both for those who enjoy the "social wing" of the gym, as well as for those who can't stand it.

For example, if you like to train alone, on your own, in silence, or with your headset, and the gym is full of guys who come to chat and give you training and diet tips that you don't want to know – you will be pissed off?

Or, at the other extreme, if you like to exchange ideas about each workout, learn about other people's diets, meet new friends, make challenges, and so on, and in your gym is each one for themselves? You won't like it either.

It is difficult, but not impossible: try to analyze the possibilities and put this on the scale!

7- Price

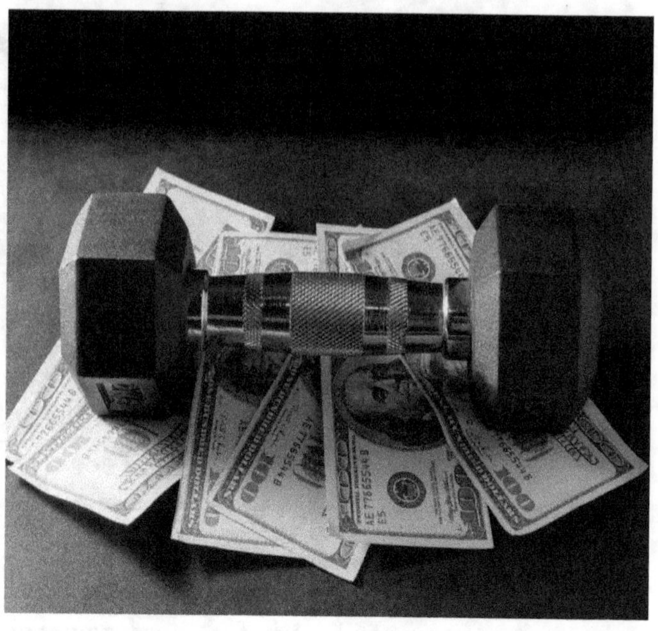

It is not possible to say that the price is the most important, but it is certainly a point to be considered.

Just don't make stupid savings: paying less and not having equipment available is an example of meaningless savings.

At the same time, the most expensive is not always the best.

The best way to assess the price of a gym is cost-benefit. And, to reach this result, the idea is to use the other six criteria mentioned above.

Do an analysis of all items, count positive and negative points of the gym in question, and, including the price on the account, you will arrive at the perfect gym for you!

Important to note: in the real world, the gym does not have to be perfect in all aspects. It needs to meet your needs!

Equipment to have at the gym

The gym may contain various simulators designed for the complex development and strengthening of muscles by performing certain movements. Some modifications provide the study of the whole body, and options for specific areas of the upper or lower mass - chest, back, buttocks, biceps, etc. Exercises on them contribute to building a figure with a beautiful relief, improving strength indicators, and mastering the correct technique.

1. THE SQUAT CAGE: YOUR MASTERPIECE

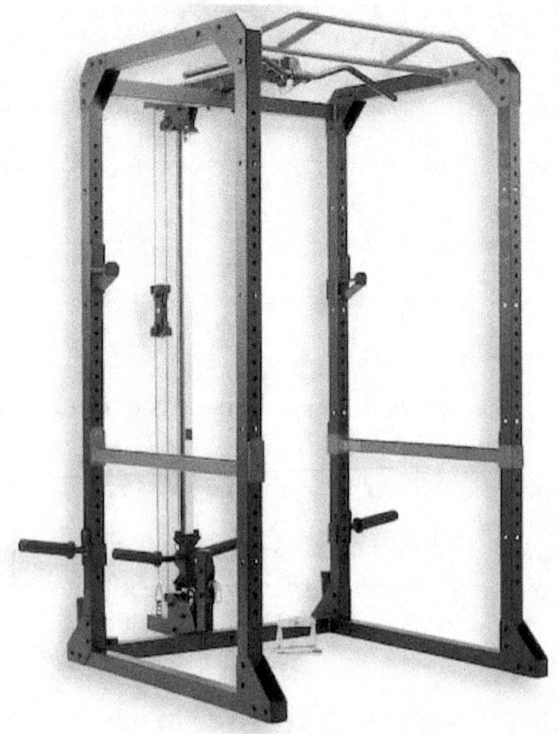

Squat cage Decathlon

- Multi-grip pull-up bar (150kg supported)
- Integrated pulley
- Robust supports 200kg of loads
- Height-adjustable safety system

It is essential and I do not want to hear anything on the subject. The squat cage is THE centerpiece of any weight room, and for good reason, it will allow you to work all your muscles. With this ultimate strength equipment, you will be able to do your squats, your bench press (adding a bench), your pull-ups, your military presses (shoulders), your bent chest pull-up, and so on ... in short, all of them. The basic exercises to gain muscle volume and burn serious calories.

Yes it is an investment and yes it can take up space but it is also durable and adaptable.

What you want on your squat cage:

- presence of safety arms (adjustable in height) to save your life and that of your back
- integrated pull-up bars (multi-grip) and dips
- an on-board pulley

2. EL CLASSICO WEIGHT BENCH

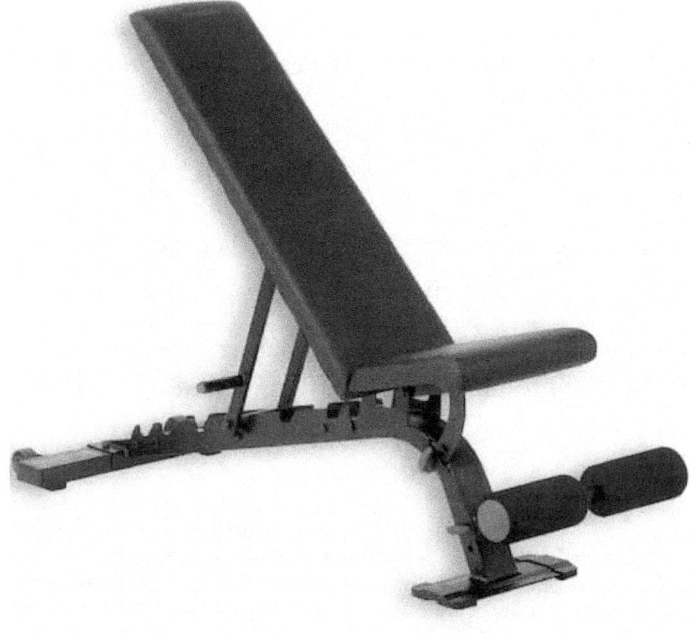

Reclining / Declining Weight Bench

- Maximum load 250kg (user + loads)
- 7 levels of inclination
- Integrated transport wheels
- Thick foam and openwork back for greater ease of movement.

"When there is the cage, there is the bench that goes with it!"

No, the weight bench is not meant to sit down to recover from your sets, at least that's not its primary interest.

Bench press with bar/dumbbells, incline, butterfly, pullover, lumberjack pull, split squat, jump squat, and so on, the bench has always been a must.

If you've gone for the squat cage you need it, the same goes if you haven't gone for the CrossFit cage, sorry.

Doing without a bench is a bit complicated, it is not replaceable, if you perform lying on the floor the exercises intended to be performed on the bench, you will not have the same range of motion, and most will not even be achievable.

We want the bench to be robust, to support the load, and, if possible, to tilt to be able to vary the working angles.

3. BARS (IRON) AND WEIGHTS

Weight bar 20Kg

- 190 kpsi
- The official length of 220cm and diameter of 28mm
- Knurling of the bar for an efficient and comfortable grip
- Rolling bar sleeves to protect your joints

We stay in the classic, but essential because you will look very smart with your squat cage without bar and weight!

And yes, the budget will increase considerably with an Olympic bar and some discs (at least 2 of 20kg, 2 of 10kg, and 2 of 5kg). Note that the official Olympic bar weighs 20kg (for men) with a diameter of 28mm on the axis and a length of 2.20m.

You want a barbell that it:

- has good quality smooth bearings
- either must have a good voltage resistance: PSI (prefer bars> 180 PSI)

Once the bar has been chosen, it's time for the weights!

They come in all sizes and materials.

You should always choose Olympic weights that are round (forget about hexagonal shapes) and if possible have integrated cuffs (a good aid for loading / unloading a bar).

Also, try to select weights that have bevels, which will help you lift a plate off the floor when it has been laid flat (without a bevel, the edge of the weight touches the floor and you cannot put your fingers in. below to pick it up).

Finally, do not forget the disc stops, I recommend this kind to you.

4. DUMBBELLS / KETTLEBELLS

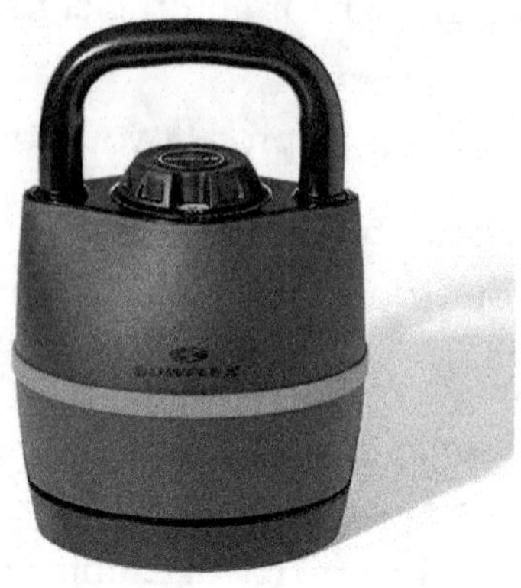

"Muscles are made with dumbbells as true as water quenches thirst."

Free weights, that's all it's true! The perfect complement to the barbell, dumbbells offer a plethora of isolation exercises.

Often they allow a greater range of motion (as on a classic bench press) and do not require having a rack at home (unlike the Olympic bar).

Also, in terms of safety, they allow you to easily drop them on the ground if you can no longer assume one more repetition, in short, a must-have!

If you're on a budget and/or little space, kick straight into a pair of adjustable dumbbells! Compact, they are expensive but avoid taking up all the space of your home gym.

In addition to the dumbbells, you should get yourself a pair of kettlebells, or even adjustable kettlebells.

While many do not consider them essential, kettlebells nevertheless allow many movements that cannot be done with dumbbells.

They, therefore, represent an interesting investment for the variety they can bring to your training programs.

Another choice is to opt for a Kettle Gryp, a nifty tool to transform any dumbbell into a kettlebell.

5. PULL-UP BAR / GYM RINGS

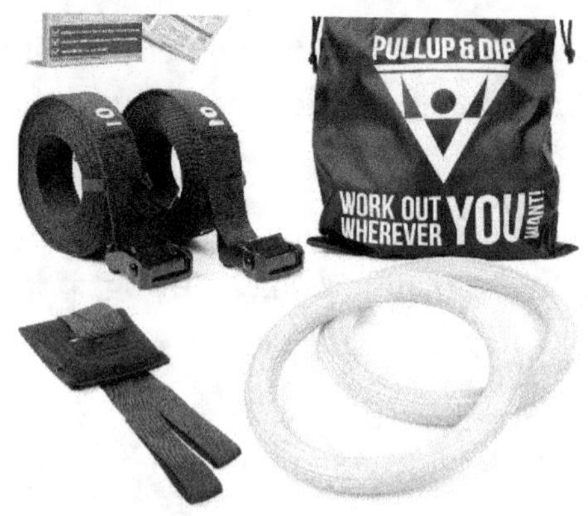

Complete Gym Rings Kit

Why this kit:

- 5 levels of resistance [2 / 7kg], [7 / 16kg], [16 / 27kg], [18 / 36kg], [22 / 57kg]
- Space-saving and accompanied by a storage bag
- Door anchoring system included
- Chalk tube included
- Quick, safe and easy assembly/disassembly

Wooden rings, pleasant to the touch

If you don't have a squat cage that incorporates a pull-up bar, then you can't do push-ups.

And it is wrong! Pull-ups are a very complete exercise that you should be able to do.

Besides the pull-up bar, you can also invest in gym rings (I highly recommend it), which can be attached to a support (squat cage or pull-up bar) at height and allow you to work on your stability.

They have the advantage of being inexpensive and very versatile.

6. PARALLEL BARS / PARALLETTES

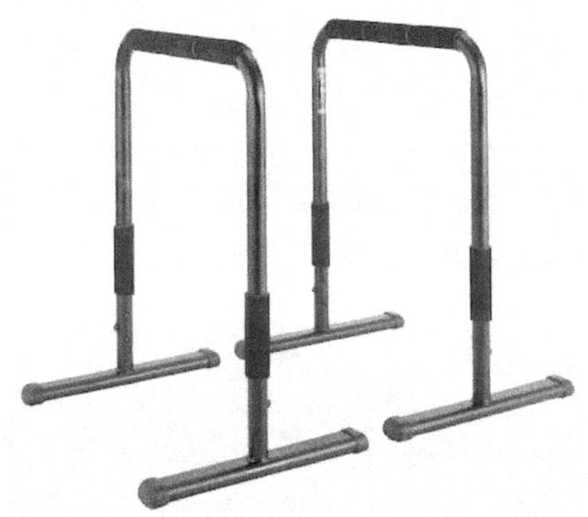

Dip bars

Why this kit:

- Resistant, support a load of 130 kg
- Small footprint, easy to store and take away.
- Thick resistant foam, compact, comfortable, and intuitive marking

One of my favorite pieces of equipment, the dip bars!

The number of exercises you can do with it is incredible! You can use it for plyometric exercises: by jumping over it, perfect for working on explosiveness, buttocks, thighs, and calves!

You can also do any core exercise, arms straight, hanging on the bars, bring your knees up to your chest, tighten your abs, and try to hold on for 20 seconds.

There are many more exercises on the list, pikes (for the shoulders) and of course the plank! If you want to impress everyone with mastering the board, you're going to have to go through this!

When the sun shines, easily carry your bars out into the garden for a vitamin D workout.

7. STRENGTH BANDS

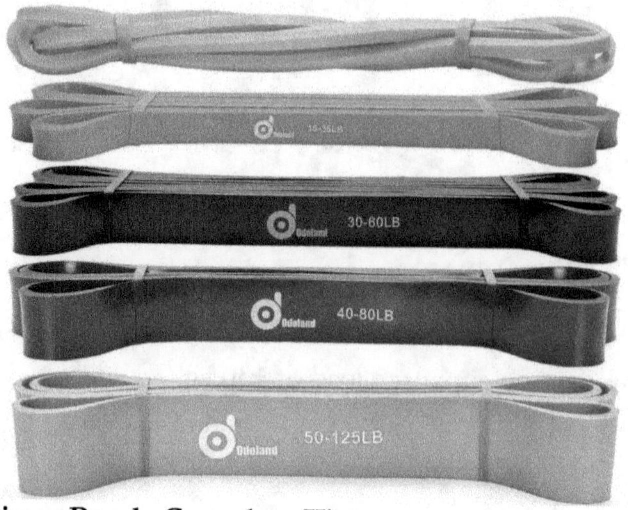

Resistor Bands Complete Kit

Why this kit: 5 levels of resistance [2 / 7kg], [7 / 16kg], [16 / 27kg], [18 / 36kg], [22 / 57kg] Space-saving and accompanied by a storage bag

- Door anchoring system included
- Handles to facilitate certain pulling exercises

Mobile, inexpensive, versatile, practical for warming up muscles or adding resistance to your exercises, elastic bands are a considerable asset for any gym!

It can be used to make bodyweight exercises very effective, but also to accentuate the work on exercises with loads, such as the famous bench press for example ... guaranteed sensations!

They will also be useful on certain stretching exercises, or to slip into a travel bag. In short, another must-have!

8. AB WHEEL

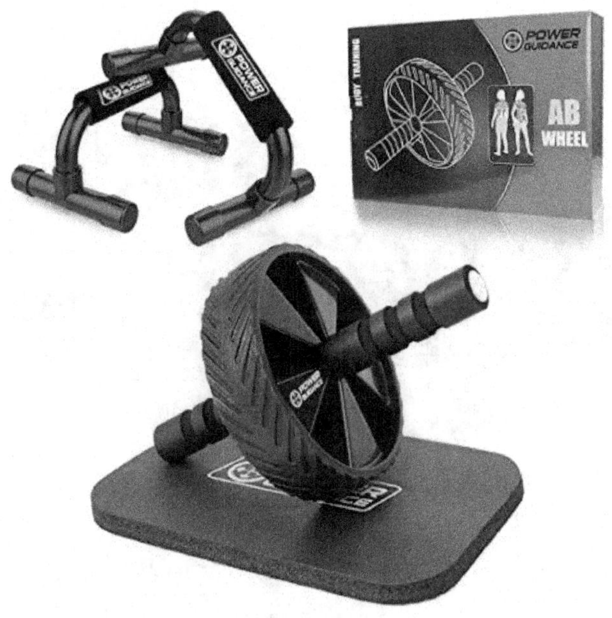

The famous, unique, ab wheel that I talk about very often. Never has such a simple tool brought me so much satisfaction for radical abdominal work!
Once again, it's up to you and your imagination to make one, it's never just a roulette wheel with a rod inside!

That's what I love so much, its simplicity, and yet, hello burns! A monster of efficiency and portability, a prominent place in the list of equipment for a home weight room for well-traced abdominal tablets!

Be careful, however, in my opinion, this is not an exercise for everyone.

9. WEIGHT BELT / WEIGHTED VEST

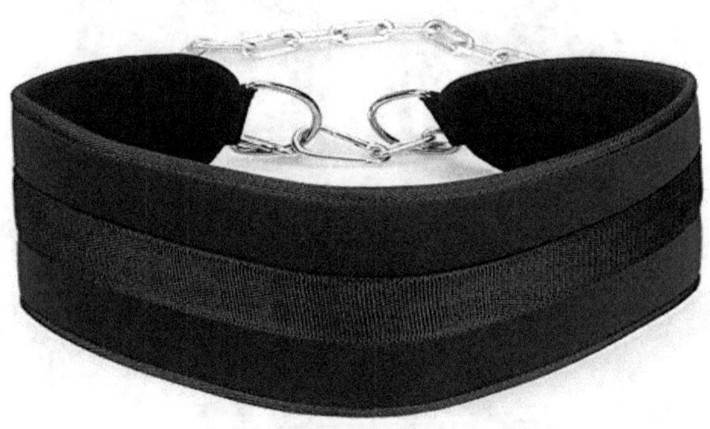

Another simple and practical accessory to turn your home into a bodybuilding sanctuary. Very simple, this belt will allow you to transform any exercise common to the weight of the body into weighted exercise.

An air squat beast immediately becomes more challenging with 20kg on the back.

Who says ballast, says more resistance, therefore more muscles! If you want to progress in pull-ups and dips, there is nothing better, you need a weight belt!

Alternative: weighted vest.

10. A SMALL BABALLE

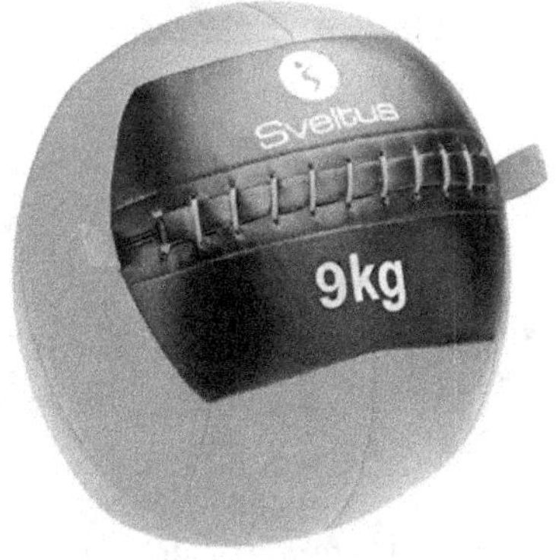

Want a gym weight room that lives up to the name? This will not happen without a bullet!

Another practical tool to increase the intensity of your gym training programs.

Workout for beginners

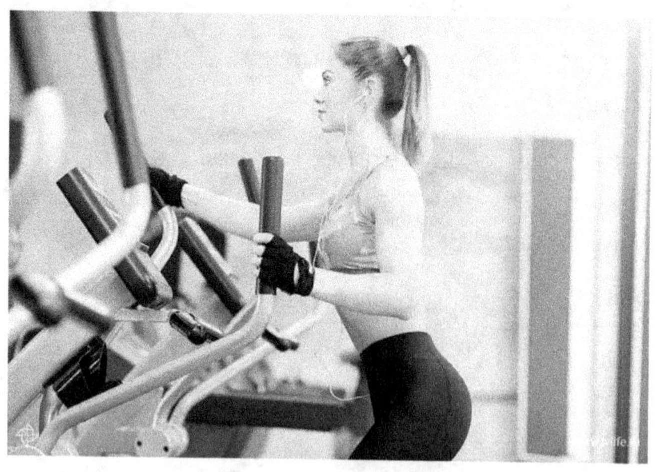

"The very first thing to do when you come to the gym is to warm up in the cardio zone. If you have any contraindications, such as problems with the musculoskeletal system or heavyweight, I recommend using elliptical trainers for warm-up. They give minimal stress to the spine, but at the same time, all muscles work.

If you prefer a treadmill, start at a low speed - 3-5 km / h, do several knee lifts, overlaps, pulling the heel to the buttock, and then gradually increase the speed to a comfortable one. Tilt angle approximately 1 ° - this tilt is equivalent to walking on an ordinary road, then can be increased to 2 °. I recommend setting the tilt to no more than 4 °. I often see how they set an incline of 6-8 ° on the track and begin to "go uphill", holding on to the handles, just to subdue it. This is a huge mistake - in this position you put a lot of stress on the joints and you will not get anything but problems and injuries after such a warm-up - you can even injure your lower back!

After warming up in this way for 10-15 minutes, you must pull the muscles: the front surface of the thigh, back, calf, ankles, muscles of the back, arms, and then you can go further, for example, into the power zone. I highly recommend going through the first lesson with a trainer, which will show you how to use the equipment correctly, how much weight, leverage to choose, etc. - your health depends on it, and besides, it is the key to a fruitful workout. "

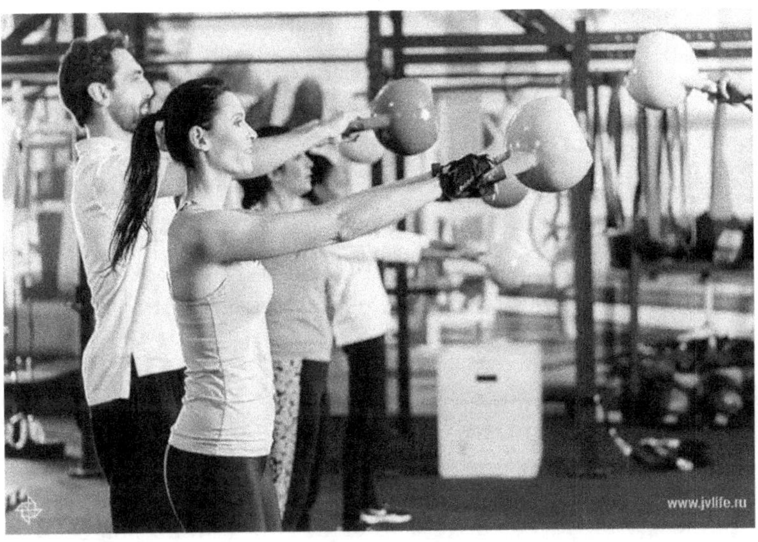

The training program depends on whether you are gaining muscle mass or want to lose weight. If you are building muscle or working out the relief, then split workouts are suitable for this purpose, when the fitness program is broken into parts and a certain muscle group is worked out every day. However, for beginners, it is better to train all muscles in one workout, but visit the gym every other day. To burn fat, add a couple of aerobic activities per week, and do strength training with low weight, with increased reps and reduced rest time between sets. Heavyweight strength training lasts about 45 minutes, and fat-burning sessions can last up to 1.5 hours.

The standard rest between exercises is 1 to 1.5 minutes.

The basic exercises for training the initial stage are the press, deadlift, and squats with a barbell on the shoulders, as well as the study of individual muscle groups. During one workout, you can do your legs (squats and lunges) and swing the press, in the next lesson it is recommended to devote time to working out the muscles of the chest and arms (push-ups and exercises with dumbbells). The third workout day is good for strengthening your back with a barbell pull to the waist, as well as exercises such as pull-ups and deadlifts.

If you have been thinking about fitness for a long time, but do not know how to work out in the gym, take a few lessons from a fitness instructor. In the future, you can practice without a coach, but at the initial stage, the beginner still needs help, which should not be neglected. This will help you exercise profitably and avoid injury.

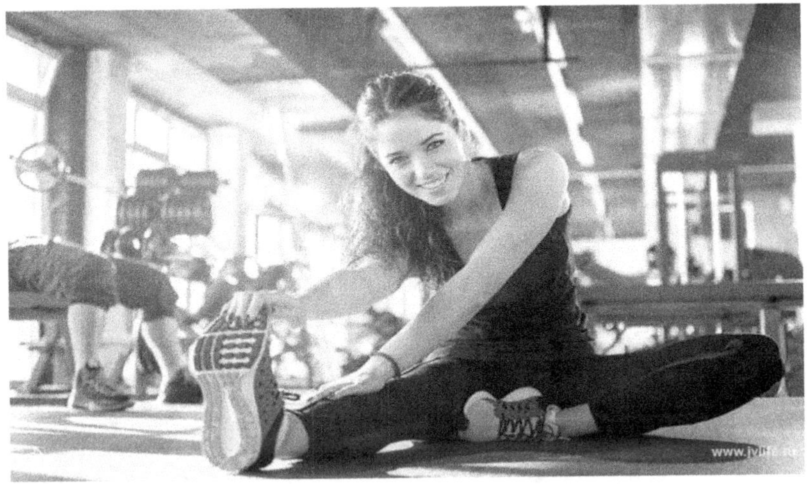

"And another very important point - never forget about stretching after a workout! Many people make a big mistake when they load their muscles during training and then forget about stretching. It is important not only for muscle elasticity, but also improves blood circulation, well-being, and functionality in your body. "

Chapter Six

A Perfect Body

First of all, to be successful in losing fat and building muscle you need to be diligent in training and watch your diet. Without these 2 basics, it will be difficult to succeed in your mission!

The success of this goal also depends on your experience: if you already practice diligently, and your muscle mass is large enough, you cannot naturally gain muscle and lose fat at the same time. It is very difficult to gain muscle and lose fat if you have already used most of your genetic potential for muscle growth.

On the other hand, if you are a beginner, then losing fat and gaining muscle at the same time is quite achievable.

Gaining muscle and losing fat are two goals that we must differentiate.

When you want to gain mass, you are programmed to eat a diet that is higher in calories than your body needs, to build muscle. On the contrary, to lose weight, you have to burn more calories than you consume.

Incompatible on paper, yes, but the body adapts well, in reality.

When it comes to training, some exercises are both good for burning fat and effective for building muscle. And the long-term effect is self-sustaining since the muscle acquired will allow you to burn more calories at rest.

The ideal will be to carry out everything written in this book, short, but intensive, made of very complete movements.

Do not forget to consume, in the hour following your session, a sufficient amount of protein, either in powder form or with a real meal.

Also, remember to hydrate yourself well. Water constitutes 70% of our body and it is essential to drink well so that all foods and supplements are properly assimilated and that the waste produced by your body is properly eliminated.

Set goals as you begin and track your progress. Keep yourself motivated that you can achieve a healthy and perfect body.

These steps will help you:

- **Step 1.** Set the rules and most importantly, follow them. It will help you to get the balance you want for your body but also to create habits to keep the perfect body during winter.

- **Step 2.** It is a mistake to set a long-term goal. Set a clear but real, short-term goal. Achieving this will increase your motivation!

- **Step 3.** As a picture is worth more than a thousand words. Keep an image that represents "your big why" and place it in a location easily visible or accessible when you need it, it will be a plus for your motivation.

- **Step 4.** Cook on Sunday for the rest of the week. This way, you won't be tempted to eat something fast (it's never healthy) because there's nothing in the fridge or you don't feel like cooking. Ah! The oven or steam cooking is always good allies for fast and healthy cooking. Eating well will make you feel lighter and more agile!

- **Step 5.** Increase the activity of your body. The key is to choose the sport that motivates you the most. The sofa is not your ally! Don't bother going for a run if you don't like it. A long walk, a morning walk, or a yoga class also helps the body get started.

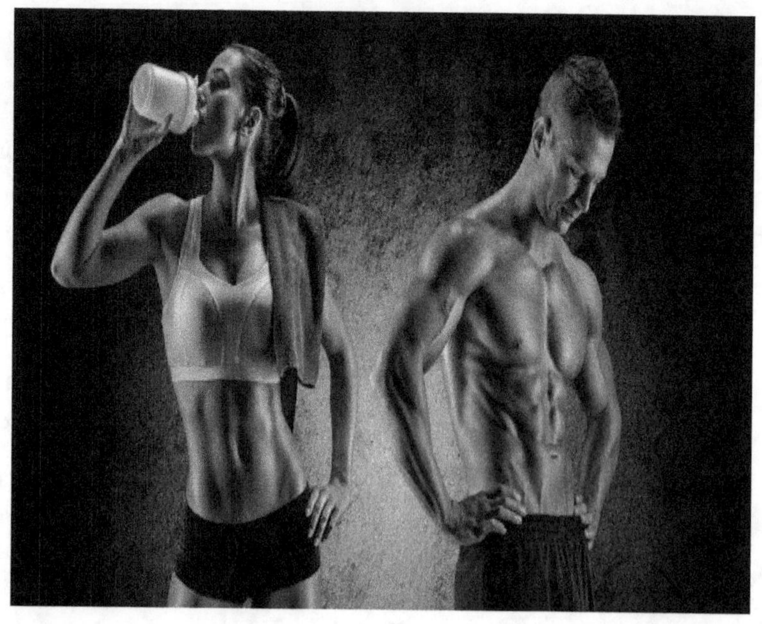

Practical tips for a continued perfect body

Now we will look at some tips that will help to maintain or even improve fitness.

1. Keep an active life. That's right. Even if you are not enrolled in a gym, try to lead a more active life, walking to work or walking with the dog.

2. Practice physical activity regularly, even if it is at least twice a week. Choose a physical activity you like and start.

3. Try to eat properly. A balanced diet, with fiber, carbohydrates, and proteins, and small fats will help a lot to keep your body weight balanced and your

energy levels adequate to practice some physical activity.

4. Make sure there is adequate rest, ensuring between 6 and 8 hours of sleep daily.

5. Adequate hydration is essential to maintain the physiological processes of an exercise practitioner. Depending on the type and intensity of physical exercise, up to 3 liters of water per day will be needed.

6. If the problem that prevents you from following a physical training plan is the lack of time, invest in more vigorous physical activities, as more intense exercises, even if practiced for short periods, increase caloric expenditure and contribute to the improvement of conditioning.

7. In your training routine include cardiorespiratory exercises (walking, running, swimming, water aerobics), muscle strength (weight training, functional training), and work on your flexibility.

8. Avoid drinking alcoholic beverages, as alcohol in the body negatively influences metabolic and physiological functions, which are essential for physical performance. Alcohol intake interferes with the absorption and use of carbohydrates, heart rate and performance, and muscle blood flow. Besides, the rate of sports injuries increases in proportion to the increase in the amount of alcohol ingested.

9. After starting a physical exercise program, control your anxiety to expect results only in the medium

and long term. In the beginning, focus on good posture during the execution of the movements, on your concentration, and have fun with your movements.

10. Exercise, preferably, with the guidance of a good Physical Education professional. This will ensure greater effectiveness and safety for you during training.

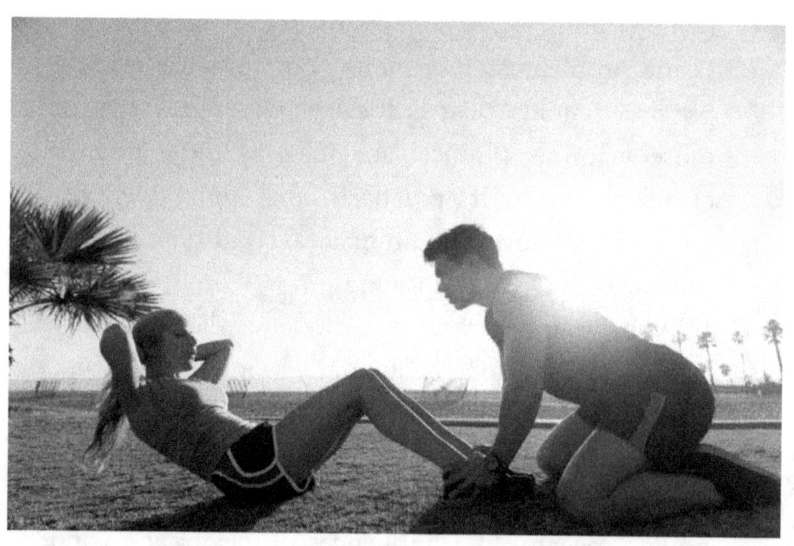

Cautions and restrictions

After becoming convinced of the importance of good physical conditioning, the individual must take some precautions during his training to increase the safety and effectiveness of the exercises.

- Warming up: Warming up is essential before all physical activities and if the weather is colder it should be done for longer and with greater emphasis. The warm-up can be organic (light walk, light trot, bicycle) or articular (rotations of the main joints). The stretching exercises light (not bending) may also be part of the heating. Every 10 minutes of organic warming, the amount of synovial fluid in the joints increases between 10 and 13%. Thus, the body is warm, flexible, the nervous system is prepared to receive a greater training load and the risk of injury falls significantly.

- Adequate clothing and footwear: It is essential to use elastic clothing that does not limit movement and whose fabric allows body sweating. Footwear should be suitable for each type of activity, remembering that sneakers must be non-slip, without loose laces, and with an anti-impact system on their sole.

- Respect for individual restrictions: Each individual carries a history, with limitations such as previous injuries, surgeries, congenital malformations, pain, and the effects of some medications. It is useless to copy a training plan made for some celebrity on the internet, as it will not suit your reality. The training should be prescribed respecting the limitations and highlighting the potential of each one.

- Hydration and temperature control: Hydrate yourself correctly before, during, and after physical exercises will guarantee the effectiveness of physiological processes, in addition to preventing hyperthermia by the heat produced during exercise. With a hydrated body, it is easier for the body to sweat and, with that, to regulate its internal temperature.

- Adequate nutrition: The body needs the energy to perform physical exercises. An individual who trains without the adequate energy supply may enter into a hypoglycemia (low blood sugar) condition, which will directly affect the functioning of the central nervous system (a system that only feeds on sugar), with low performance and, in more severe cases, it may even lead the individual to a coma. Post-exercise nutrition is also very important, as the body that exercises need a lot to replace its proteins, a fundamental nutrient for the formation of muscles and bones.

- Guidance from a good professional: It is always worth remembering that to perform good physical training, adapted to your specificities and limitations, a good Physical Education professional will make all the difference. It will greatly increase your chances of obtaining better results with the training, in addition to offering security during the execution of the movements.

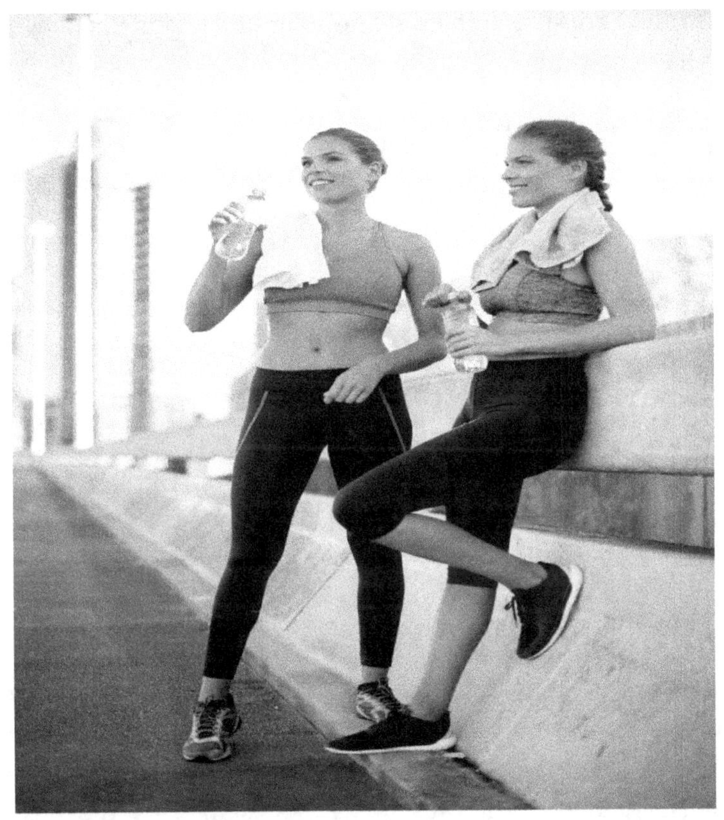

The importance of having a perfect body

A sedentary lifestyle is a major cause of death and health problems in the world. In this scenario, you need to know the importance of physical exercise within the routine to have a healthier and more balanced life.

Best of all, it is not necessary to spend hours inside the gym to have a better quality of life. It is possible to gradually introduce physical activity sessions until the body gets used to the new routine.

1. Disease prevention

Physical activity decreases the risk of developing cardiovascular disease. That's because, by putting the body in motion, the body produces a high-density lipoprotein (HDL), known as "good" cholesterol, which reduces bad cholesterol and decreases the level of triglycerides in the blood.

This improves blood flow and reduces the risk of heart disease, in addition to preventing stroke (stroke), metabolic syndrome, type 2 diabetes, arthritis, and even some types of cancer.

2. Controls blood pressure

You can opt for simple activities, such as running, biking, walking, swimming, climbing up and downstairs. Aerobic exercises are the most recommended by doctors. This regular practice promotes greater resistance of the heart and reduces blood pressure and the risk of heart disease.

3. Increases muscle strength

The continuous and lasting effort contributes to the strengthening and toning of the muscles. Soon, in a few months, you realize that you have gained muscle strength and that the musculature is more apparent. Physical activity also contributes to injury prevention; exercises focused on weight training are usually the most recommended by doctors.

4. Improves sleep quality

The body needs to sleep approximately 8 hours a day to maintain its organic functions healthily. In this sense, the practice of physical exercise directly contributes to reducing the risk of insomnia and controlling restless legs syndrome, since the movement of the body controls circadian cycles (it works as a kind of biological clock).

Thus, if you usually suffer from insomnia and other problems while sleeping, the ideal is to practice physical activities in the morning or the afternoon. Therefore, the body will release endorphins during the day and you will feel more energetic and energetic. In turn, if you prefer to exercise at night, opt for a lighter activity to avoid insomnia since right after physical activity people tend to become more alert and active, which makes sleep difficult.

5. Controls the weight

Having a fit body is one of the greatest goals of those who exercise. Regular physical activity contributes to the loss of body fat, reduces excess weight, and prevents obesity and diabetes. This is because, when moving the body, you burn calories (and the more intense the rhythm of the exercise, the greater the burn).

In this sense, running is an excellent option for those who want to lose a few extra pounds. However, it has a strong impact and is perhaps not the most suitable for those suffering from joint and tendon problems. In these cases, the ideal is to opt for a light walk, swimming, or exercise bike.

Anyway, the practice of physical activities is directly related to a balanced diet. Therefore, weight loss will only be effective with the adoption of a healthy diet.

6. Improves the quality of breathing

Breathing is also strengthened through physical activity. It is recommended that you inhale through your nose and breathe out through your mouth, which prevents you from getting short of breath during exercise. By strengthening the respiratory system, there is less risk of bronchitis, asthma, and other respiratory diseases.

7. Increases the feeling of happiness

During the practice of physical exercise, the body releases important chemical substances, such as dopamine and serotonin, which are hormones that promote the sensation of pleasure and well-being. They help to have greater control over emotions.

Over time, you will notice an improvement in your mood and will experience happier and more pleasant days, in addition to having more motivation to perform routine tasks. Therefore, the risks of developing symptoms of depression, stress, and anxiety are lower.

It is important to mention that depression and other emotional and psychiatric problems must be properly treated with medical monitoring. Physical exercise serves as an adjunct to assist in treatment but does not replace the work of the psychologist or psychiatrist.

8. Improves flexibility

The exercise helps the practitioner to develop greater flexibility. Therefore, include a few moments of stretching before, during, and after physical activity. This care is important since elasticity helps to strengthen tendons and ligaments, reducing shortening problems and improving the performance of daily tasks more easily.

9. Promotes socialization

The practice of group physical exercises is a way to meet new people and be more motivated to continue training; it is an excellent opportunity to socialize and make new friends. You can choose to work out at a gym and take group classes or find groups that practice classes outdoors, such as squares. Also, there are exercises for children, which allow you to do family activities.

Knowing the importance of physical exercise is essential to avoid the risks of a sedentary lifestyle and live healthier. The benefits of moving the body have already been proven by science. There are many options for activities, from a simple walk to swimming, to weight training and other sports. So you have no excuse for not moving!

"The key is in the balance of body and mind"

Being aware, mainly, and performing a series of steps will allow you to achieve results quickly, but above all effective. We promise you! Take a piece of paper and pencil, and note that the most important thing is to choose daily routines that, in principle, will be easy to perform.

Moreover, if you organize yourself, and above all, if you have the will, it is as if it was done.

You too can have a perfect body!

Healthy Body Q&A's

Why is physical activity so important for my health?
Regular moderate physical activity is one of the simplest ways to improve and maintain your health. It has the potential to prevent and control certain diseases such as cardiovascular disease, diabetes, obesity, and osteoporosis. Being physically active increases your energy level, helps to reduce tension, and lowers cholesterol and blood pressure levels. It also decreases the risk for some cancers, especially colon cancer. Regular physical activity promotes the healthy growth and development of children and young people. It increases confidence, self-esteem, and feelings of accomplishment; older adults benefit both from healthy habits throughout their lives and from recent changes in physical activity. It is important to age in a healthy way, improves and maintains the quality of life and independence. Daily physical activity helps people with some type of disability, improving mobility and energy levels. It can also prevent or reduce certain degrees of disability.

What do you mean by "physical activity"?

Physical activity is any movement of the body that results in an expenditure of energy (calories). Simply, move! When you take a brisk walk, play, skate, clean the house, dance, or climb a ladder, you are moving towards health.

How much physical activity do I need to improve and maintain my health?

Any amount of physical activity will make you feel good. The minimum amount of physical activity required for disease prevention is approximately 30 minutes of moderate activity daily. For people who count calories, this translates to approximately 150 calories per day. However, you can search for Health without counting calories. The formula is simple: at least half an hour of moderate physical activity each day. This may mean getting off the bus two stops before on the way to work, for a 20-minute walk and one-stop before returning home to walk for another 10 minutes.

Ten minutes of cleaning the house twice a day plus 10 minutes of cycling. A 30-minute basketball game or dance with your brothers, sisters, friends, or children. If you are starting physical activity, you can start with a few minutes of activity a day and gradually increase your stride and reach up to 30 minutes. Remember that half an hour is only the minimum recommendation. Of course, the more time you spend "Moving to Health", the more you will profit.

The most important thing is to move!

Is it possible to lose weight and never put on weight again?

Getting fatter depends on several factors, as well as losing weight too. There is no magic pill that makes you thin forever and that will never put you back on weight, regardless of your habits. I am sorry for this, but it is the truth.

We know that some people really have a very fast metabolism and even find it difficult to gain weight and who exclude themselves from this rule, but they are the exception and not the majority. Although many studies are being done even in the field of genetic engineering to arrive at a product that provides this same "skinny forever" effect to everyone, science is a long way from achieving this. So for now there is no way. If you leave the line for a long time, you can get back to fat. I always say that sustainable weight loss promotes a change in behavior and mentality through dietary reeducation. And this is the secret to never putting on weight again: stay faithful to this re-education. If the mind changes, the body follows, and then you don't put on weight again, but it is a condition of action and reaction: if the head remains fat, the body will follow, and then you don't put on weight again, but it is a condition of action and reaction: if the head remains fat, the body will follow, because the habits will go in the opposite direction to promote weight loss.

How do I determine the intensity of my physical activity?

"Intensity" is relative; the same activity may need more effort if done by a new practitioner than if done by someone who has been exercising regularly for some time.

In general, your perceived exertion rate is a very accurate measure of the intensity level.

Here are some additional guidelines that will help you determine the level of intensity of your activity:

Your intensity level will be low if you can speak, sing if your breathing is even and you are not sweating.

Your intensity level will be moderate if you can speak, but you cannot sing if your breathing is rapid and deep and if you are sweating after 10 minutes.

Your intensity level will be high if you can speak short phrases, but you cannot sing if your breathing is very fast and deep and if you are sweating after 3 to 5 minutes.

How long should I exercise for?

There is no need to start with a heavy load of exercise, start slowly.

Shorter periods of exercise can provide the same benefits as longer sessions.

Starting slowly will also help you avoid injury and burnout.

What is the recommended amount of exercise?

The most recent recommendations from the American College of Sports Medicine and the American Heart Association are that you should exercise for at least 30 minutes at a moderate intensity five days a week or for 20 minutes at a high intensity three days a week to preserve health and reduce the risk of chronic diseases.

When you reach your final weight goal, your goal will be to generate 4 to 6 Active Points per day - this is the amount considered effective to maintain your weight loss.

To start, however, you should try to generate 1 to 3 Active Points per day.

Is it better to work out in the morning?

It is worth exercising at any time of the day. The time of day does not matter.

Is it true that if I am not losing weight, it is because I am gaining muscle?

The weight is the same for 500 grams of muscle and 500 grams of fat.

However, 500 grams of muscle has less volume (that is, takes up less space) than 500 grams of fat.

If your weight loss is not going as you want, but your body looks more toned and your measurements are smaller, then you are experiencing a muscle increase due to physical activity. If the weight remains the same and you are not getting more toned and with reduced measures, it is because physical activity is not influencing your weight loss process.

Why do men and women lose weight differently?

Men and women tend to lose weight differently based on the types of fat they contain and the factors to get pregnant. Weight loss has less to do with your body's natural shape and more to do with genetics, how your hormones work, and your metabolism.

References

American College of Sports Medicine. Position Stand: Appropriate Physical Activity Intervention Strategies for Weight Loss and Prevention of Weight Regain for Adults. Medicine & Science in Sports & Exercise, 2009.

Bendahan D, Mattei JP, Ghattas B, Confort-Gouny S, Le Guern ME, Cozzone PJ. Citrulline/malate promotes aerobic energy production in human exercising muscles. Br J Sports Med.

Bucci L, Lm U. Proteins and amino acid supplements in exercise and sport. In: Driskell J, Wolinsky I, editors. Energy-yield macronutrients and energy metabolism in sports nutrition. Boca Raton: CRC Press; 2000. p. 191–212

Calder PC, Yaqoob P .. (1999). Glutamine and the immune system .. Amino Acids. 17 (3), p227-241.

Cullen KW, Zakeri I. 2004. Fruits, vegetables, milk, and sweetened beverages consumption and access to à la carte/snack bar meals at school. Am J Public Health 94(3):463–467.

Daura Abadia De-Souza, Lewis Joel Greene, Pharmacological Nutrition After Burn Injury, The Journal of Nutrition, Volume 128, Issue 5, May 1998, Pages 797–803, https://doi.org/10.1093/jn/128.5.797 2002 Aug; 36 (4): 282-9.

Esposito K, Pontillo A, Di Palo C, Giugliano G, Masella M, Marfella R, et al. Effect of weight loss and lifestyle changes on vascular inflammatory markers in obese women: a randomized trial. JAMA 2003; 289 (14): 1799-804.

Goldstein ER, Ziegenfuss T, Kalman D, Kreider R, Campbell B, Wilborn C, Taylor L, Willoughby D, Stout J, Graves BS, Wildman R, Ivy JL, Spano M, Smith AE, Antonio J. International society of sports nutrition stand position: caffeine and performance. J Int Soc Sports Nutr. 2010; 7 (1): 5.

Graham TE. Caffeine and exercise: metabolism, endurance, and performance. Sports Med. 2001; 31 (11): 785–807

Harris RC, Tallon MJ, Dunnett M, Boobis L, Coakley J, Kim HJ, Fallowfield JL, Hill CA, Sale C, Wise JA. The absorption of orally supplied beta-alanine and its effect on muscle carnosine synthesis in human vastus lateralis. Amino Acids. 2006; 30 (3): 279–89.

Hoffman JR, Ratamess NA, Faigenbaum AD, Ross R, Kang J, Stout JR, Wise JA. Short-duration beta-alanine supplementation increases training volume and reduces subjective feelings of fatigue in college football players. Nutr Res. 2008; 28 (1): 31–5

Ivy JL, Kammer L, Ding Z, Wang B, Bernard JR, Liao YH, Hwang J. Improved cycling time-trial performance after ingestion of a caffeine energy drink. Int J Sport Nutr Exerc Metab. 2009; 19 (1): 61–78.

Jager R, Kerksick CM, Campbell BI, Cribb PJ, Wells SD, Skwiat TM, Purpura M, Ziegenfuss TN, Ferrando AA, Arent SM, Smith-Ryan AE, Stout JR, Arciero PJ, Ormsbee

MJ, Taylor LW, Wilborn CD, Kalman DS, Kreider RB, Willoughby DS, Hoffman JR, Krzykowski JL, Antonio J. International society of sports nutrition position stand: protein and exercise. J Int Soc Sports Nutr. 2017; 14:20

Jakicic JM, et al. American College of Sports Medicine Position Stand. Appropriate intervention strategies for weight loss and prevention of weight regain in adults. Med Sci Sports Exerc.2001; 33 (12): 2145-56, 2001.

Kreider RB. Effects of creatine supplementation on performance and training adaptations. Mol Cell Biochem. 2003; 244 (1–2): 89–94

Oliveira, TFB, Laterza, MC, Ferreira, R., Werneck, FZ, Paizão, JA, & Coelho, EF (2011). Effectiveness of a physical exercise evaluation and prescription program for women. Brazilian Journal of Health Sciences, 9 (30), 1-8.

Olsen S, Aagaard P, Kadi F, Tufekovic G, Verney J, Olesen JL, Suetta C, Kjaer M. Creatine supplementation augments the increase in satellite cell and myonuclei number in human skeletal muscle induced by strength training. J Physiol. 2006; 573 (Pt 2): 525–34

Paes, Santiago T. et al. Metabolic effects of exercise on childhood obesity: a current view. Revista Paulista de Pediatria. 2015; 33 (1): 122-129.

Paes, Santiago T., Bianchini, Renato M. Childhood Obesity: Role of Non-Pharmacological Program of Body Weight Reduction Treatment. J Endocrinol Diabetes Obes 3 (3): 1077.

Paes, Santiago T., Bianchini, Renato M. How to Start an Exercise Program for Obese Individuals and Minimize the Incidence of Orthopedic Problems? JJ Obesity. 2015. 1 (3): 021.

Paes, Santiago T., Bianchini, Renato M. Obesity: How can Interventions Ensure Treatment Success? Int J Endocrinol Metab Disord 2015, 1 (4): 15:21.

Pérez-Guisado J, Jakeman PM. Citrulline malate enhances athletic anaerobic performance and relieves muscle soreness . J Strength Cond Res . (2010)

Phillips SM, Chevalier S, Leidy HJ. Protein "requirements" beyond the rda: implications for optimizing health. Appl Physiol Nutr Metab. 2016; 41 (5): 565–72

Phillips SM, Van Loon LJC. Dietary protein for athletes: from requirements to optimum adaptation. J Sports Sci. 2011; 29 (Suppl 1): S29–38.

Pollock, ML et al. Med. Sci. Sports Exerc. 1998; 30 (6), 975.

Rodrigues, AJD (2013). The benefits of regular physical exercise as a contribution to the quality of life. Federal University of Rondônia Foundation Health Center.

Rohlfs, ICPM, Rotta, TM, Luft, CDB, Andrade, A., Krebs, RJ, & Carvalho, T. Brunel's Mood Scale (BRUMS): Instrument for the early detection of overtraining syndrome. Brazilian Journal of Sports Medicine, 2008, 14 (3), 176-181.

SANTOS, M., and others. The effects of interval training and continuous training on the reduction of body composition in adult women. Revista Virtual EFArtigos (Natal), v.2, n.23, p.3-12,, April 2005

Shimomura 1 Y, Inaguma A, Watanabe S, Yamamoto Y, Muramatsu Y, Bajotto G, Sato J, Shimomura N, Kobayashi H, Mawatari K .. (2010). Branched-chain amino acid supplementation before squat exercise and delayed-onset muscle soreness. International journal of sports nutrition and exercise metabolism. 3 (10), p236-234.

SILVA, CA; LIMA, WC Physical exercise to improve the quality of life of individuals with insomnia. Movement, Rio Grande do Sul, vol. 7, n. 14, p. 49-56, 2001.

Smith AE, Walter AA, Graef JL, Kendall KL, Moon JR, Lockwood CM, Fakuda DH, Beck TW, Cramer JT, Stout JR. Effects of beta-alanine supplementation and high-intensity interval training on endurance performance and body composition in men; a double-blind trial. J Int Soc Sports Nutr. 2009; 6 (1): 5.

Sureda A, Córdova A, Ferrer MD, Pérez G, Tur JA, Pons A .. (2010). L-citrulline-malate influences over branched-chain amino acid utilization during exercise .. Euro Journal Of Applied Psychology. 1 (1),

Tipton KD, Witard OC. Protein requirements and recommendations for athletes: relevance of ivory tower arguments for practical recommendations. Clin Sports Med. 2007; 26 (1): 17–36.

Tipton KD. Nutritional support for exercise-induced injuries. Sports Med. 2015; 45 (Suppl 1): S93–104.

Tsiros MD et al. Cognitive behavioral therapy improve diet and body composition in overweight and obese adolescents. Am J Clin Nutr 2008; 87: 1134–40.

U.S. Department of Health and Human Services and US Department of Agriculture. Dietary Guidelines for Americans, 2005. 6th Edition, Washington, DC: US Government Printing Office, January 2005.

Volek JS, Duncan ND, Mazzetti SA, Staron RS, Putukian M, Gomez AL, Pearson DR, Fink WJ, Kraemer WJ. Performance and muscle fiber adaptations to creatine supplementation and heavy resistance training. Med Sci Sports Exerc. 1999; 31 (8): 1147–56.

Werneck, FZ, & Navarro, CA Level of physical activity and mood in adolescents. Psychology: Theory and Research, 2001, 27 (2), 189 -193

Werneck, FZ, Bara Filho, MG, Coelho, EF, & Ribeiro, LCS (2010). Acute effect of type and intensity of exercise on mood states. Brazilian Journal of Physical Activity & Health.15 (4), 211-217.

Wiles JD, Coleman D, Tegerdine M, Swaine IL. The effects of caffeine ingestion on performance time, speed, and power during a laboratory-based 1 km cycling time-trial. J Sports Sci. 2006; 24 (11): 1165–71.